SURGEON & LOVER

FULFILLMENT & FOLLY

MICHAEL M. MEGUID MD

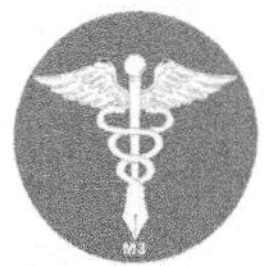

The events and conversations in this book have been set down to the best of the author's ability, although some names and details have been changed to protect the privacy of individuals.

ISBN 978-0-9992988-2-4

M3 Scientific Media
Marco Island, Florida 34145, USA
www.michaelmeguid.com

Cover image: Daria Dyk - Shutterstock

PRAISE FOR SURGEON & LOVER

Surgeon & Lover: Fulfillment & Folly is the captivating story of a young man struggling with nearly incapacitating injuries left by damage inflicted by parental neglect and a rootless childhood. Meguid compensates with driving ambition and a need for love to give him the equilibrium and self-justification he needs. Told with honesty, self-deprecation, humor, and literary artistry, it is the portrait of a lonely man, making sometimes inappropriate decisions in his emotional vulnerability. We can't help but admire how he faces surgery and life head-on as he works tirelessly in his profession to help others. We root for him all the way. Though third in the quartet *A Surgeon's Tale,* this biographical sketch can stand on its own.

—Jan Tramontano, author of *The Me I was with You*

Other Works by Michael M. Meguid MD

A SURGEON'S TALE: FOUR PART SERIES

Spanning nearly ten decades, from 1930's onward, momentous and dramatic social changes occurred. *A Surgeon's Tale* is a historical biographical series, the fecundity of medical tales, that reaches beyond the merely personal to convey something of the cultures, people, politics, and places that touch the inscrutable heart of human nature. This multifaceted journey percolates with diabolic tales of intrigue, coldly detached scientific dishonesty, sensual medical discoveries, succulently passionate illicit romance, unspeakable merciless scoundrels, and devious ascetic murder all the while disclosing the rites, rituals, rules and language of surgery. It is a story of life with all its warts, betrayal, love and affection—or lack of it, but ultimately, it is a story of persistence, endurance, triumph and passion.

Volume I. ***Root & Branches: A Family Saga Like No Other***

Nobel laureate, Elie Wiesel once wrote, "God made man because He loves stories." And when a story is told by a master story-teller, we, His creatures are likewise enamored. *Roots & Branches* is one such tale. Before we even finish the first chapter, a harrowing account of a near fatal heart attack in a cab stuck in a traffic jam in New York City, we are hooked. We just *know* that we are going to enjoy savoring every page, but simultaneously aware that the book is only 322 pages long.

In his dedication, Meguid writes, "... to Victoria, who couldn't have known her man for he didn't know himself." So perhaps, this biography was his attempt to find out who he was, and why, and to invite his readers to join in his quest.

He introduces us to his father, an Egyptian, who was a brilliant scholar, warm and charming, but frequently absent and who died when Meguid was nearly 12 years old. His mother, a German, was incapable of showing any affection, which left deep emotional scars, while his older sister, furious about being usurped by her younger brother, was jealous and hostile. *Roots & Branches* moves from Egypt, where the young Meguid thrives in his Egyptian extended family, enjoying laughter-filled sumptuous Friday meals, to war torn post-war Hamburg with his stern grandparents, where boiled turnips, cabbage and pork belly meals were eaten in silence. A few years later, Meguid is taken to cold, rainy Manchester, then finally back to Cairo again. Throughout these years, he had to continuously adapt to different cultures while witnessing major political events.

There are many delights in this amazing biography which I will leave to you to discover. However, what I find amazing about *Roots & Branches* is despite all the challenges and heartaches that Meguid faced, his innate optimistic spirit and intelligence enabled him to rise above them.

And finally, what a wonderful gift Meguid has bequeathed his children, grandchildren, and more. I ended up feeling that I would have loved it if my father or mother had written a similar book. I would have liked to really *know* them.

—Mona Ateek, Professor of English,
American University Cairo, Egypt

"A frank and richly described account of a surgeon's childhood." —*Kirkus Review.*

Volume II. ***Mastering the Knife: Seeking Identity & Finding Belonging***

Mastering the Knife reaches beyond the purely personal to convey something of the people, period, and places that made the author. Working sometimes like a memoirist and sometimes like an anthropologist or ethnographer, he lifts a veil on the rites, rituals, rules (written and unspoken), and language of medicine, especially surgery.

Meguid is a masterful storyteller, and the story that he seems to have lighted on is about the peculiar mixture of temperament, intellect, skill, circumstance, discipline and luck that go into the making of a remarkable life. Some powerful forces are arrayed against him, of course: racism and xenophobia as well as parental cruelty, neglect and abandonment. The author gets a lot of narrative momentum from the sense of pushing against the forces—even the ones inside his own head—agitating for defeat and failure.

Scenes capture the drama of a particular moment in very few words. Much of the dialogue is crisp. Sometimes it's laugh-out-loud funny. Whenever the author turns his descriptive powers on a place—whether landscape or structure—the writing turns vivid and evocative. Much of the prose about the practice of medicine or surgery, as seen through the eyes of a student, is precise and memorable. The reader finds herself being educated through Meguid's eyes.

—Jennifer Brice, Associate Professor of English, Colgate,
author of *Unlearning to Fly*

Volume III. ***Surgeon & Lover: Fulfillment & Folly***

Surgeon & Lover is a brilliant and very personal expose of a life first bridging two national, social and language cultures, then absorbing what is best from a third culture, that which is scholarly and academic. It can be argued that this mix largely contributed to a vision and a universal language reflected in the author's success as a doctor and surgeon of the highest quality.

—Patricia Sands, bestselling author of the
Love in Provence series

MAKING THE CUT PODCAST

Overcoming a childhood of abandonment and neglect, Dr. Meguid becomes a world-renowned surgeon. But before that he had to learn to become a man. Now, that story is revealed.

makingthecutpodcast.com

Dedicated with gratitude to:

Robin S. Pilcher FRCS FRCP (1902–1994), Professor of Surgery at University College Hospital, who enthusiastically encouraged my interest in surgery when I was a medical student.

WG Austen MD FACS, Professor of Surgery, Harvard Medical School, Chief of the Surgical Service, Massachusetts General Hospital, who facilitated my coming to Boston.

Frances D. Moore MD FACS, (1913–2001), Professor of Surgery Harvard Medical, Chief of the Surgical Service, Peter Bent Brigham Hospital, Boston who enabled my surgical training in the U.S. thus changing my life.

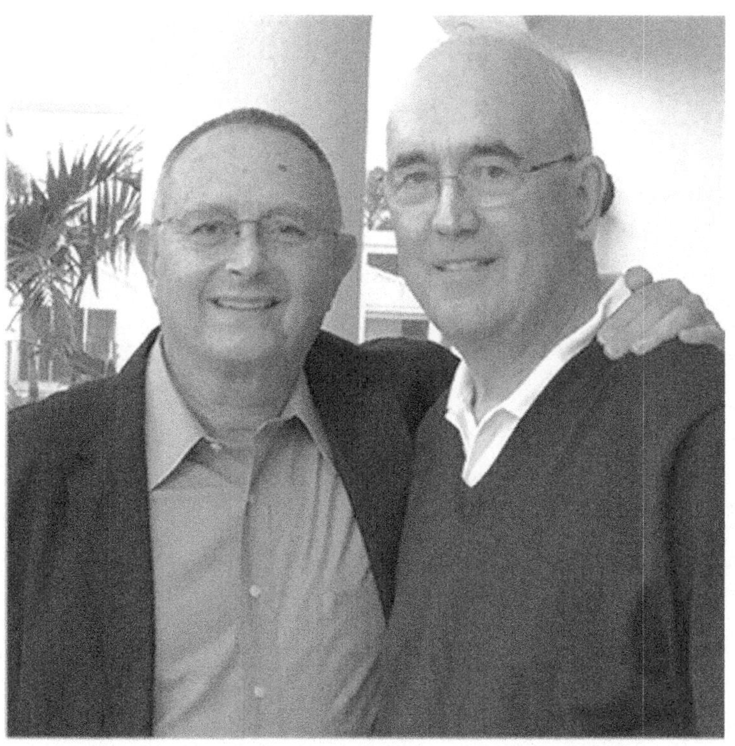

Rory McCloy BSc MD FRCS, the captain of our 1963-64 University College London eight crew and Michael M Meguid MD PhD MFA FACS. In honor of our 55-year friendship. Marco Island 2018.

Art is a lie which helps us see the truth
—Albert Camus

There are lovers' content with longing.
I'm not one of them.
—Rumi

CONTENTS

AUTHOR'S NOTE

Similar to events in *Roots & Branches* and *Mastering the Knife*, the first and second volume of the quartet, entitled *A Surgeon's Tale*, the occurrences in this sequence are as I remember them and are inspired by factual events. Memories formed in association to traumatic events are remembered sharper than general memories. Narrative techniques are used in telling this story to convey some characters and scenes which are composites.

Certain experiences, which occurred over fifty years ago, are enriched by personalities—some colorful, others disreputable, have been reordered. The happenings in *Surgeon & Lover: Fulfillment & Folly* took place at a time when social behavior, social expectations, and mores were very different from those of current times. The names and identifying characteristics of some individuals have been changed to protect them; as unique individuals, however, they may discover themselves in these pages. In other cases, I used names in accordance with historical facts and records.

I've endeavored to be as authentic as possible, relying on my personal archives, a journal, letters, and photo albums.

Quotes from letters originate from correspondence. Whereas when written over fifty plus years ago, some letters fell into the private domain and were never intended to see the light of day, the beauty, passion and tenderness of their message especially in the era of text messages raises these letters to the realm of poetry and merit sharing with the reader in the relevant context. This account does not attempt to tell the whole story. Others may recall things differently or have their own versions of what transpired.

British Medical Education in the 1960s

Requirements
High/Grammar School: 2–3 years (biology, chemistry, physics; Bachelor Medicine) Burnage Grammar School, Manchester ⟶ 1st MB

Medical School/College
2 years basic science. University College London ⟶ 2nd MB

3 years Clinical Training plus, University College Hospital, London
⟶ MBBS

(MBBS is given by the General Medical Council of the United Kingdom.)

One-year Compulsory Internship
6 months medicine. House Physician (HP) Bethnal Green Hospital
6 months surgery. House Surgeon (HS) Royal Ear Hospital, UCH

(A student can stand in for Locum HP or Locum HS for HP or HS when they take a compulsory two-week holiday)

Receive a medical license issued by General Medical Council of the United Kingdom to practice as GP or to start specialized training.

Steps to specialize as a general surgeon in UK in the 1960s
Become a Fellow Royal College Surgeons (FRCS).

Study for 6–12 months. Basic science (anatomy, physiology pathology) *as it applies to the surgical patient.*
Sit and pass primary exam given by Royal College Surgeon
⟶ **Primary FRCS***

3–4 years surgical training as Surgical Registrar (Residency)
Sit and pass final exam given by Royal College Surgeon
⟶ **Final FRCS***

*FRCS is equal to the American College of Surgeon's FACS

PROLOGUE

When I was growing up in Egypt, Germany and England surrounded by elders who controlled and managed me in accordance with *their* cultural norms, I often felt confused about the conflicts inherent in their mores. I used to think that one day, when I was an adult, I'd no longer have these problems. The "me" would be the one who decided my response to life's events. I wish it was true. Seeking and understanding the "me" is an old-aged endeavor; the Roman poet Virgil, born 70 B.C., pondered in his famous poem *The Aeneid*, "Who am I, and why?"

Egyptians, British and Germans approach life quite differently. As an adult I've struggled with the burden arising from three conflicting societal expectations and responses, the "fitting in" that we all strive for in life. The bundle on my back contained these influencers—characteristics that competed to express my true self and followed me around wherever I went. They thrived on validation and love. Their nemesis is loneliness and its accompanying pain.

The infuriating thing was that I accepted this burden as a

natural part of me. I could slide with ease into different societies until I was confronted with the common human trait of someone wanting to categorize me—to put me into a box that fitted *their* life's experience, *their* norms. At that point my identity became a question to me. One of the personas would determine how I responded, sometimes resulting in the opposite outcome of what the situation expected—both comical and sad.

Many years have passed as I voyaged through school, early romances and relationships. Nothing was simple. My baggage was always imprinting every situation. In hindsight these feelings stemmed from the wound of abandonment in early childhood.

I see identity as two parts of an equation: our inherited DNA and the very personal "how" it is expressed. As I grew older, to circumvent my demons I buried myself in my chosen work, invested in the care of patients, was drawn to the need of others, all the while buttressed with love from my stoic wife. But at any time, the outcome of this internal struggle was fragile.

Many of the conflicting feelings that arose were re-lived while writing both *Roots & Branches* and *Mastering the Knife.* The latter had an appropriate subtitle of *Seeking Identity & Finding Belonging* precisely because as I moved from child to empowered young adult these feelings became more acute and like Virgil, I sought their answer. The current story, *Surgeon & Lover: Fulfillment & Folly*, and my other books in the series *A Surgeon's Tale* became part of a therapeutic odyssey to understand who is the authentic "me." The Italian football striker, Mario Barotelli, is quoted to have said, "Some say abandonment is a wound that never heals. I say only that an abandoned child never forgets."

In a seminal paper published by Dr. Judith Herman in the *Journal of Traumatic Stress* in 1992, followed by her book *Trauma*

& Recovery, she described a psychological trait in adults that resulted from prolonged trauma in childhood, trauma from which they cannot escape because it is inflicted on them by the person or situation that they experience. This emotional or physical trauma wreaks havoc to an infant, child and young adult's brain development and the formation of basic personality characteristics and leaves its imprint on brain and body. It is now identified as Complex—PTSD. I could well have been one of Dr. Herman's subjects, thirty years before she labeled and codified the adult consequences of childhood abuse and trauma. As a teenager and young adult well before 1992, I *lived* some of the symptom complex: trust, anxiety, concentration, acceptance and shame, among other symptoms. No wonder these topics appear throughout my memoirs including *Surgeon & Lover: Fulfillment & Folly.*

Others, too, have suffered similar early childhood experiences. It is estimated that twenty-five percent of the American population—some fifty million people—have symptoms of Complex—PTSD. Included in this category are abandoned children, those living in foster homes, those adopted, children who grew up in dysfunctional families, those who grew up in families where there was alcohol or drugs abuse, family violence and sexual abuse. I consider myself lucky for, relatively speaking, I had a "normal" childhood life.

Lastly, symptoms have been recognized in dogs and cats. Certainly, my beloved Lucy was abandoned, beaten and terrorized as a pup. After I adopted her from the Naples Humane Society, Florida ,when she was about eighteen months old, it took Lucy about eighteen months to not cower before me. Our daily therapy was love and positive reinforcement. Yet to this day, some ten years later, she becomes withdrawn and worried when I leave the house, despite my telling her of my intent to return. The welcome I receive on my return is that deserving of a king. The rest of the time I'm never out of her visual site. We are most suited.

Against my childhood odds I managed; forging myself into a surgeon/scientist, husband and father. I grew to accept myself, and even tolerate the "me" I uncovered. Veracity is and was crucial to recognize the reality I faced and lived, and which molded me over my life-time—an asset to a surgeon. Yet it is a commodity that often makes society and individuals uncomfortable. By embracing our failings and recognizing our truths, it buttresses a genuine human and on a greater scale the triumphs and failures of the human story. It does not detract from the habitual seeking of "lovability." Ultimately, I hope you will find the series of books in *A Surgeon's Tale* as a tale of self-discovery, determination, persistence, triumph and passion.

PART I

BOSTON & ANTIGUA

WINTER 1967

I come from a long line of storytellers and this is my inimitable tale.
—Unknown

1

TEMPLE ON FRUIT STREET

Massachusetts General Hospital is hardly general.
Aphorism

Wearily, I plunked my suitcase on the unmade bed by the window in Vanderbilt Hall, Boston. I would pay $16 per week and an additional $1.25 a week for linen rental service. I was surprised to see another bed in the corner, with baggage slipped under its metal frame. With whom was I sharing a room? Exhausted and jet lagged, I made my bed and gladly fell into it fully clothed. There was no last thought as I escaped into a deep sleep.

I joined a group of about twenty people congregating outside the Emergency Room (ER) entrance to Mass General Hospital on Fruit Street at 5:45 a.m. I was quite conspicuous in my gray suit while the rest of the surgeons were in white.

There were two teams of residents: the White Service for private patients and the Ward Service for indigents. The senior resident, Everett Sugarbaker, directed me to the second group where the medical students introduced themselves. Dr. Levin, the team leader, explained the routine we would follow. The welcoming friendliness and my immediate inclusion were entirely different to the reserved, hierarchical British system from which I had come.

Rounds began in the ER, where we identified overnight surgical patients awaiting a semi-urgent operation—the "add-ons." These patients came to the ER with surgical problems and were subsequently worked up by ER residents during the night. Dr. Levin agreed they were in need of an operation.

From the ER, we rode up the elevator to the intensive care unit (ICU). The ICU concept was entirely new to me. About twenty bays distinct from the nearby operating suites were staffed with specially trained and dedicated nurses for the most seriously ill surgical patients who needed specialized care and close monitoring "24/7"—an American idiom I immediately understood.

Our first patient that day left a lasting impression. Mr. Renaldo was a recent Italian immigrant, who was unconscious and suffered from hemorrhagic pancreatitis—a condition I had never encountered. Intubated and paralyzed, the relatively young patient had an open abdominal wound extending from the xyphoid at the lower sternum to the pubis, covered by large, moist gauze pads to keep his guts from spilling out. There was a tube in every orifice—a nasogastric to drain stomach, bile, and GI juices, a Foley to empty the bladder, an arterial catheter to monitor blood pressure, a central venous catheter to draw blood, and one to input saline into the abdominal cavity, with a sump suction to drain fluid output.

Dr. Sugarbaker must have seen me grow pale. He explained that in hemorrhagic pancreatitis, the digestive juices were attacking its organ. There was no definitive or curative treatment; they washed out the destructive enzymes in the hopes of ending the cycle. Earlier, he had used a sterile teaspoon to scrape out dead pancreatic tissue. I learned that binge drinking had caused the patient's condition.

The effort, energy, and cost invested in trying to save one human being with a self-inflicted illness amazed me. I realized that in this situation, medical care and treatment decisions were not influenced by moral judgment or hopelessness. These complicated and challenging surgical problems were approached with a resolve to overcome them. The overwhelmingly upbeat attitude impressed me. Such a work ethos was pervasive and infectious, and I felt free of the constraints of tradition and I could thrive in this positive atmosphere—the eagerness and the can-do approach to surgical problems.

Mr. Renaldo consumed an enormous amount of our time. I was not sure if he would recover, but he did serve to draw together my disparate physiological knowledge acquired at University College Medical School, London. I began to appreciate that in this unconscious man, who was covered only with a cotton sheet and surrounded by life-support machinery, the sum of the physiological parameters—temperature, pulse, respiration, blood pressure, fluid status and level of consciousness—painted the picture of his condition. Standing by his bedside, I understood that God had to be here in his fullest presence for Mr. Renaldo to make it—an awareness or prayer I would revisit many times in my surgical career.

One duty on the medical student's scud list was to calculate Mr. Renaldo's daily fluid status because he could not compensate for his losses by drinking water. The patient's twenty-four-hour fluid intake had to equal his output, with additional fluid to offset losses from the skin, increased evaporation occurring with each one-degree of temperature rise, and losses from the open abdominal cavity. The change in daily body weight, although crude, was an integrator of these calculations. The details made my head spin. A summary of these figures was part of the daily presentation of the patient's status during morning and evening rounds. Despite such fine-tuning of patient care, over time, Mr. Renaldo developed anasarca—the general bloating of his body with swelling of his brain. I was overwhelmed by the complexity of managing such a patient, the likes of which I had never seen at the Whittington or even at University College Hospital. I was there when, after almost thirty-six days, Mr. Renaldo finally succumbed.

A separate, specialty-trained trauma team managed the ICU's trauma patients, whose all-encompassing care was beyond my grasp in the initial days for lack of exposure to this discipline during my training. Despite my "greenness," doing rounds and being available at all times to assist on trauma operative cases gave me the opportunity to integrate my basic science knowledge and begin to apply this to pre- and post-operative care, an aspect poorly understood by me up to then. Operating was a skill that improved with time, but it had to stand on a solid foundation and understanding of basic science—the knowledge of how the body worked as was drummed into me in the first two years of anatomy, physiology, biochemistry and so on in preparation for the second MB at University College, London.

Thereafter, we started rounds on the ward service. These patients did not have an attending surgeon and often lacked insurance; they were the responsibility of the chief resident, who was in his fifth year of general surgical training, but who had access to senior surgeons—attending staff—for guidance and consultation. A student would present their patient's progress during the night, with the intern chiming in to provide the latest developments or additional data, such as the results of tests. I noticed a professional camaraderie, an attitude of mutual help, regardless of the level of training. The stress of the surgical situation and the common goal of wanting to help patients survive forged solidarity among the different levels of staff, nurses and students. The sicker the patient, the more the common concern among the group, and the more the individual group members expressed the emotional responsibility, all of which was strikingly different from the pecking order in England.

A glaring distinction from rounds back home was that the nurses did not accompany us. Orders were written into a book, flagged by patient name, which a secretary transcribed, freeing the nurses from administrative work. I had my doubts as to the efficiency of this system, for I much preferred the nurse's presence on rounds. The advantage was that one could hear the nurses' professional opinions concerning patient progress and communicate directly to them the changes that were wanted. Throughout the rounds, the intern made scud lists of tasks for those students not assigned to the OR that day.

After the group dispersed, we went to the cafeteria. I had my first meal since arriving in America. Sitting together, we divided up our workload. Next to me was Tom Sos, who lived near Vanderbilt Hall. He generously offered to pick me up and give me a ride with him to and from the hospital. On the days when the operation where I was assisting went into the late evening, he suggested I could sleep in the on-call room. He was interested in becoming a radiologist. The other students eating breakfast were very welcoming, friendly and helpful.

I was unaccustomed to being on a first name basis from the moment I met someone, let alone to their nicknames. A jovial student introduced himself as Stu, short for Stuart. You would never call anyone "Stu" in London! Jan Breslow was a tall, broad-shouldered and handsome fellow with a particular interest in the hyperlipidemias, while Edith, a quiet individual, planned to become an internist or psychiatrist. Since I was the only one seriously committed to surgery I could assist with as many operations as I wanted—an operative feast for me. Our obligations included admitting and working up assigned patients and, like in London, attending mandatory morning and afternoon teaching seminars for those not scrubbed.

I was impressed by their visionary paths for the future. Mine was relatively ambiguous. I wanted to become a surgeon but had no idea how I would make this happen. At that time in England, training and upward mobility depended in part on a more hit-or-miss approach. Promotion to consultant or professor took longer to achieve, more due to the filling of "dead man's shoes." Did this fit in with my imagined short life expectancy? Since my Daddy dropped dead from a massive pulmonary embolus while he was a patient at the American University Beirut at fifty, I irrationally feared my life span would end at the same age. Whatever I wanted to achieve had to be done by then, putting a sense of urgency in my life.

The American system of surgical residency was more straightforward. After completing medical school, graduates entered a surgical residency program of their choice and underwent systematic training for a specific number of years. On completing residency, one sat for the American Board of Surgery exam, following which one started a practice. The concept was appealing to me—a bit like being back at school—as there were measurable landmarks.

Despite my jet lag, I went to Dr. Gerald Austen's office to sign in and announce my presence. His friendly secretary welcomed me and gave me a key to an on-call room and food coupons—limited to $2 per day—usually used for breakfast. Dinner was free after the refectory formally closed at 11 p.m., when we could eat whatever leftovers were available.

She told me that one of the surgeons, Dr. George Nardi, had invited me to his home for Thanksgiving dinner in three weeks —a very kindly gesture that I accepted. She added that I *could* participate in the students' oral surgical test, which was done in early December. She further suggested that I might want to read Dr. Nardi's surgical textbook and added that the end of the rotation would be December 15, 1967.

"Friday, December 15?"

"Yes. You know, Christmas break. Why?"

"Well, no one told me. My return ticket to London is on December 30."

She saw my consternation. "You can always go skiing in Vermont, or to the beach in Miami," she said, and focused her attention on her work.

What would I do in freezing Boston, alone for two weeks, and where would I live? It would cost a pretty penny to change to an earlier return flight, even if I could get a seat during the Christmas season on my inexpensive London-Boston round-trip ticket.

The image I had seen in BOAC's flight magazine popped up: vacationing on the island of Antigua. It was not the £60 excursion fare from New York to Antigua that caught my eye but the accompanying scene. An aerial view of green palm trees, branches hanging over a yellow beach lapped by a turquoise blue sea. A romantic young couple lay sunbathing on a large red towel. My thoughts went to my darling Victoria. .I wondered if such a holiday would interest her, for she, too, had time off at Christmas. I was concerned that it might not seem proper to Victoria's mother to have her unmarried daughter gallivanting about a Caribbean playground with a man. The rumor would fly around the very conservative village of Sea View on the Isle of Wight, or as we called it, the Isle of Serenity. Of course, Shirley, her mother, had a good idea that we were sleeping together, if not at 95 Gower Street, then when I spent nights with her daughter in her flat at Ladbroke Grove, Notting Hill. On the surface, my German family would probably frown upon it, too, and it was certainly taboo in Egypt.

Despite the liberating cultural shift in American sexual attitudes happening at this time, I wanted the semblance of decency and respectability, perhaps because I now felt the responsibility that came with working in the highbrow surgical world in Boston.

Victoria and I had discussed marriage before I left. Perhaps we could get married in Boston; the last two weeks of December were a perfect time to honeymoon before returning to London when our busy schedules would resume. Shirley could arrange a fancy wedding reception after I graduated in May.

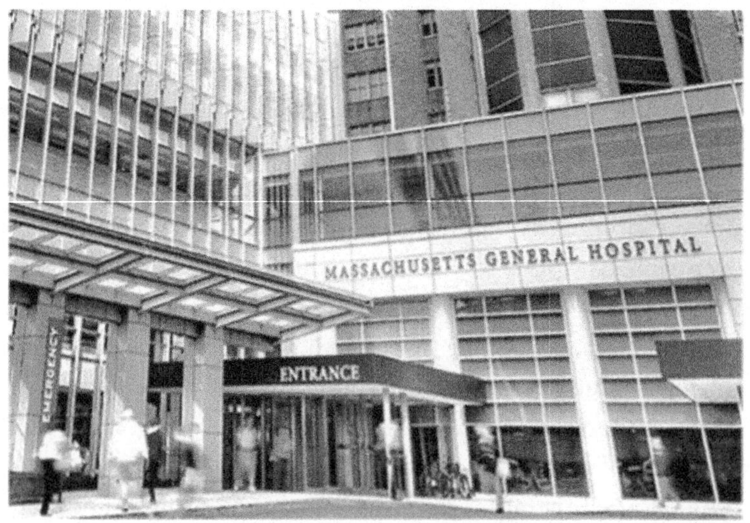

Courtesy of Massachusetts General Hospital

The rest of the ward rounds that first day were a blur, given my jet lag and difficulty in understanding the numerous American medical acronyms. The patients here were sicker than I was accustomed to seeing and presented with more advanced stages of their illnesses; not to mention, the operations performed were more complex and sophisticated. I had difficulty understanding the various stages of a disease and found myself drawing on my physiological knowledge to follow the proposed therapy. Not only were the acronyms so different from the ones I had learned in London but they were more colorful and frequently used, often drawing on Spanish. It would take me a few days of intense attention to catch onto the new lingo and still longer before I found myself using it with comfort and confidence.

The next day, we were finishing rounds when all the residents' pagers went off simultaneously. "Code Blue ER" squawked repeatedly from an overhead intercom. The team took off like a stampeding herd down the stairway. I was not sure what was happening but followed to catch up with them on the pavement outside the ER door. A blur of white dressed bodies stooped over a man on a gurney.

One of the physicians was pumping the patient's corpulent chest with vigor, shouting out orders for meds. With focused intensity, a nurse drew them up from her cardiac cart. She handed a syringe to the team leader, who stuck the long needle straight through the undershirt into the patient's heart. As the resuscitation continued, the body lifted an inch off the gurney with each forceful thrust.

Another resident frantically tried to start an intravenous line. Nurses attempted to cut off the man's trousers, while others pushed the gurney into the building. I was a helpless bystander, never having witnessed or learned to participate in a cardiac arrest, which made me acutely aware of how much I had to learn. An ambulance, a fire engine with flashing lights, and two police cars surrounded the scene. I noticed that all the first responders spoke with a peculiar Boston accent—or was it an Irish brogue? The firefighters refused to leave their colleague on the gurney.

The effort continued in the ER, with the patient surrounded by police, nurses, and residents. They intubated and oxygenated him. They stripped him naked and hooked him up to monitors. He looked so pale and young, with waxen facial features. After thirty minutes, the enthusiastic effort to save his life ebbed. With no response from the patient to drugs, external cardiac massage, intra-cardiac stimulant and defibrillation, the attempt ended as if stipulated in a textbook exercise, and they pronounced him dead.

The nurses pieced together the story. The deceased had visited his girlfriend while her husband was attending church. During intercourse, he experienced chest pain and lightheadedness. Fearing a scandal, she dressed him, which explained the misaligned buttons on his shirt and his poorly fitting trousers. She clothed him in his winter coat while he was floating in and out of consciousness, losing valuable time before she telephoned his friends at the fire station, trying to keep matters confidential instead of dialing 911—the American number used in emergencies.

The resident team drifted away from the lifeless body. We left a chaotic scene of syringes, blood, catheters and clothes strewn on the floor, presumably for the nurses to pick up. The mood was a somber one of reflection and defeat. The usually upbeat, can-do spirits were slowly draining like water out of a sink. I wondered about the effect of repeated patient failure on a surgeon's psyche over a lifetime.

By walking away to attend to life we avoided the awkward conversation brought on by grief suffered by the surviving loved ones. As physicians we avoided dealing with this vital half of life, becoming used to it but hopefully not blasé to the death of our patients. In my subdued state I understood the proclamation that he was dead—he was now organic matter—lifeless like my cadaver Fred whom we dissected during anatomy class. As a subtext to life the team dealt with death, yet he was now of no particular interest in the hectic surgical day. I said a silent prayer for the patient and his survivors for there was no time to linger in the spiritual realm.

Nevertheless, the French surgeon Leriche's saying that every surgeon carries within him a small cemetery, where from time to time he goes to pray—a place of bitterness and regret—where he must look for an explanation for his failures, haunted me.

The low energy state among our team lasted only until Dr. Sugarbaker called us to order and reminded us of our tasks for the day—some to assist in the OR, others to the wards. I was to help Dr. Hermes Grillo, a thoracic surgeon I met at the scrub sink. We dipped our arms into a vat of alcohol up to our elbows—a sterility method I was sure would soon catch on in England. We toweled off, and the nurses dressed us in sterile paper gowns and gloved us, all while Dr. Grillo was relating pleasant memories of the various times he had spent as a surgical resident in England.

Unlike in London, the patient was rolled into the OR awake and only after Dr. Grillo greeted him was he put to sleep. My London brain imagined that this practice extended the turnover time between cases.

Dr. Grillo was reconstructing a man's trachea—the windpipe—located at a high level in the neck between the jaw and the sternal notch above the thyroid gland. The tracheal rings had been damaged several months earlier when a tube for an emergency tracheostomy had been inserted during an emergency resuscitation. It had saved the patient's life. As it healed, it narrowed the main airway, making it progressively more strenuous for the patient to breath.

After washing down the patient's neck and draping it, Dr. Grillo handed me the scalpel. I made a skin crease neck incision above the old scar with the intent to dissect out the old craggy scar. Grasping the scar tissue with a clamp, he raised it to assist my continued resection of the skin and its underlying fibrous tissue. A fresh bleeding plane of the neck was entered. I could see what had to be done next: dissect down to the tracheal rings, resect the damaged old ring, and mobilize the entire trachea to obtain vertical mobility such that the new tracheal ends could be sewn together again. This was beyond my current surgical skill. But watching Dr. Grillo do it would eventually allow me to emulate the operative procedure.

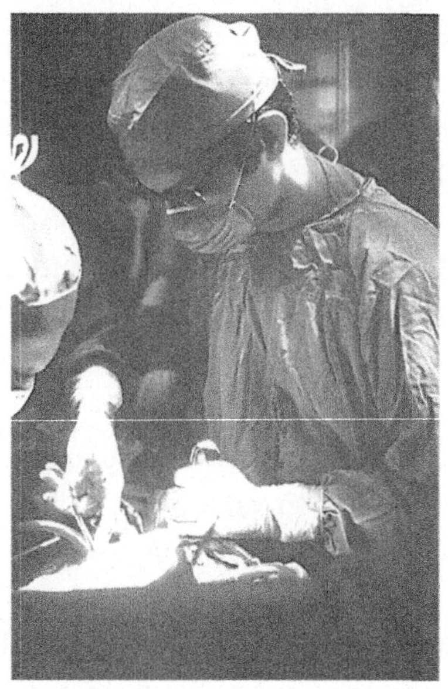

"You did that elegantly."

Taking a new scalpel, he proceeded. I felt a sense of usefulness and pride in my ability to assist him.

He opened the neck, exposed the trachea, and excised the damaged ring, giving a quiet blow-by-blow description of what he was doing while he mobilized the rest of the trachea in the chest, freeing it from its attachments to the surrounding lung tissues. He reconstructed the continuity of the windpipe by sewing together the upper and lower sections. I held the skin retractors to give him the exposure he required and ensured his operative field was as free of blood as possible. He knew I was a medical student from London, yet he sensed I was not a novice at the operating table. He told the scrub to give me the needle holder, which was preloaded with a small size chromic suture for closing the deep layer of the skin, telling me to start in the middle of the wound and to divide the remaining wound sections in half. This ensured that the wound would be closed evenly. He cut the suture above the knots and then showed me how to close the subcuticular layer of the wound with a single running stitch that closed this layer, approximating the skin with steri-strips to result in a fine-looking hairline incision. The nurse then placed a firm dressing over the wound.

While we were closing, he told me that he had built an entire career on reconstructing tracheas and excising tumors involving the windpipe. He had trained generations of surgeons in his techniques and had designed several surgical instruments specifically for these operations. I marveled at the strategy—learn a specialty, such as thoracic surgery, while focusing narrowly on an organ and becoming an expert in its care. I was awed by the proficiency needed to reconstruct a human windpipe—to restore normality for the patient.

Another professor I frequently scrubbed with was Dr. Paul Russell, who performed kidney transplants. Once more, the very concept of extending a person's existence and restoring their normal life through surgical intervention greatly impressed me. My horizons were expanding.

Reluctantly, I was drawn into a vascular emergency procedure. The vascular service's chief resident, a man with seven years of surgical training, and his crew of fellow residents wheeled in a middle-aged patient with an embolus that had lodged in the main artery of the leg. There were no measurable pulses in the foot by Doppler ultrasound, and the appendage was cold and white. I had nightmarish flashbacks of the evening of UCH's annual Christmas Ball a year earlier, when I was stuck in theater assisting on my first vascular case. Mr. Hart was poorly prepared, the operating room and the X-ray facilities were not optimum for such a complex vascular situation and the timing of the operation, on the eve of a major social event that engaged most of the faculty, was a poor choice. And the outcome . . .

At Mass General, the operating room was well equipped for vascular surgery, having overhead X-ray equipment worked by a radiology technician, who was also in the room. The appropriate instruments and specific sutures were available. Once the patient was asleep with his groin prepped and draped, the femoral artery was dissected out. Despite my dread, this operation was different.

The chief resident placed special vascular clamps above the artery to prevent hemorrhaging when he made a small cut into it. He passed a vascular catheter down the leg. Once the overhead X-ray scan showed its opaque tip was beyond the suspected clot, he inflated a small balloon and slowly pulled back the catheter into the incision, returning clotted red blood and a denser white embolus. I could hear the echo of blood flowing in the distal arteries, as measured by the Doppler, and the leg almost immediately pinked up.

He placed the embolus on a green towel that covered a side table, and there was a general buzz of "ah ha" among the residents. I missed the significance of this crucial piece of evidence. There was an air of satisfaction in the room as the chief resident carried the specimen off to the lab, leaving his juniors to close the wound.

The pathology report, ready that evening, showed the white embolus to be myxoma tissue. It could have originated from a tumor of the heart because seventy-five percent of myxoma tumors occur in the left atrium, the small chamber sitting on the ventricle. I now understood the triumphant "ah ha." I spent time reading about the condition in the library, waiting for the cafeteria to close to the public so that I could freely gorge myself on the day's leftovers.

A few days later, the heart-lung pump team stood by, ready to help divert the blood from the heart after they cracked open the patient's chest. The uniqueness of the case drew a crowd of spectators, who stood three-deep to watch the operation. On walking in, I first met my benefactor, Dr. Gerald Austen. After a very gracious and welcoming introduction, he placed me on a stack of stools to observe the procedure over the heads of the crowd. Once the patient was on the heart-lung machine and the heartbeat had stopped, the tension in the room rose as his resident opened the left atrium and cleared it of blood. A beautiful, delicate, sea anemone-type tumor, a few millimeters in size, grew on the cusp of the mitral valve. There were no other tumors. With the élan of a perfect golf swing, the surgeon swiftly cut the tumor off the mitral valve cusp to a crescendo of cheers. It was my first time observing open-heart surgery. I felt faint, stumbled off the stools into Dr. Austen's arms, and embarrassingly blacked out.

Mass General was the mecca of surgery in the Northeast and drew difficult cases. The complexity and spectrum of surgical diseases and the numerous feats of operative skill left me in awe. The level of eagerness among the residents and my fellow medical students was astonishing. Their dedication to surgery and teaching was impressive, and their resolve for patient care was like nothing I had seen before. There was an atmosphere of enthusiasm and a willingness to extend the boundaries of surgical knowledge, free of the constraints of tradition or rank.

Despite my admiration and respect for British traditions, I was fast becoming addicted to the vitality, the "can-do" attitude, that surrounded me in Boston.

2

LIFE AS A SURGICAL STUDENT

A chance to cut is a chance to cure
—Anonymous

The wind was biting, and the heavy clouds discharged snow nearly every day. Initially, the sight of white magic floating down from a heavily laden sky captivated me, reminding me of the enchanting time I first saw snow in Wedel, Germany, when I was four years old. This mid-November snowfall did not let up. Huge snowplows with flashing lights barreled past the hospital, shoving snow to one side and spraying salt.

Outside, the world grew eerily quiet, and in the muted night, there was a smattering of traffic and a twinkling of streetlights. It took me a while to realize that veterans of prior snowstorms had slipped away. I found myself nearly alone in the warm hospital and was stranded when a state of emergency was declared and public transportation ceased.

I lived three days and nights at Mass General, seeing the same staff faces on the wards and in the corridors. Patient admissions for routine operations dried up, as did the supply of blood to the blood bank. The cafeteria no longer served fresh fruit. The staff in the cafeteria, too, was stuck in the hospital. They soon recognized me—pale, tired, unshaven and starving, wandering in between cases. I questioned how fresh the food was because they allowed me to choose dishes, even at lunch, without asking for a meal ticket. What I missed the most was a decent cup of British tea: boiling water poured over loose-leaf black tea in a teapot and served with milk. Disliking the severe cold weather, I never once set foot outside the building. By early afternoon the next day, the sun came out, converting the snow and slush into thin layers of black ice as the storm receded.

Emergency admissions increased. Ambulances deposited critically ill elderly patients in the ER starting at around 5 p.m. I assisted in operations for perforated gastric and duodenal ulcers. Driving was hazardous, and a deluge of trauma patients from motor vehicle accidents appeared—which was new to my surgical experience. By 8 or 9 p.m., motor vehicle accidents were replaced by a wave of gunshot wounds, which ended sometime after midnight. I had not previously encountered such disruption of human anatomy—blunt injuries in motor vehicle accidents or penetrating wounds from gunshots. Certainly, guns were not a part of the British social fabric. My volunteering to assist was welcome since there was a limited number of residents. I came to admire the breed called the Trauma Surgeon. They operated swiftly, in every body cavity, not only salvaging patients but frequently snatching their patients from the jaws of death.

I was seduced by the dynamic and systematic approach to the early management of a trauma patient. I was in awe of what could be done and what was done to save patients' lives. Since I was not part of the trauma team, I did not assist with operations or postoperative care and was merely an observer.

Many of the techniques applied to the management of their patients were developed during the war in Vietnam. Although I had no time to read the paper, the deaths and casualties of the war were a daily discussion among the few residents at meals, whose status was a deferral from conscription. I remembered my anxious time in Cairo during the battles with Israel and my aversion to meaningless death and destruction.

The faculty appreciated my zest for work, encouraging and reinforcing that element of my personality. Unlike in England, where eagerness is understated and matters were approached with an air of reserve and subtlety, expressing enthusiasm in America was not disdained. The last time I had enjoyed such euphoria, such a feeling of being alive, was when I was learning to glide.

Each week, every complication and death was reviewed in front of the entire surgical faculty at the morbidity and mortality conference. During these meeting a resident presented a synopsis of the patient's illness, the operative techniques used and the complications encountered. The faculty discussed different aspects of the case with the intent of learning from mistakes made. If the patient died, the pathologist projected the post-mortem findings. General discussions followed. The five categories of complications Professor Pilcher at University College Hospital had mentioned to me—errors in diagnosis, operative technique, patient management, clinical judgment, and those due to patient's disease—were assigned and became meaningful, given the context of our discussions. I wondered if Professor Pilcher had attended such a meeting.

I learned more than surgery, for I saw grown men—surgical residents—reduced to a state of regret and even self-deprecation when things went wrong. I also witnessed redemption and human growth, as regret grew into a second chance—magnanimously part of the American psyche.

Finally, more like the traditional tutorial format in London, there were regular teaching meetings on general surgical topics, where I found I had an edge on the clinical knowledge of disease and its pathophysiology.

The ambitious drive I inherited from my father could be fulfilled, unencumbered by the accident of my birth and buttressed by my acceptance as a human being and surgeon; my zebra stripes of dark and white, of Egyptian and German heritage, were not visible. Among many fellow medical students, I was an equal. I thrived in this atmosphere and wondered if getting my surgical training in America might be possible.

3

LOVE'S STRESS TEST

Love is our true destiny.
We do not find the meaning of life by ourselves alone—we find it with another.
—Thomas Merton

Was I ready for marriage? It was a recurring and vexing question. I missed Victoria more than anything. My love for her made me feel alive even though we hadn't had the necessary free time to develop the mature love that forged cohesive bonding. The thought of her constantly invaded my mind when I wasn't consumed by reading about the upcoming surgical procedure, preparing for an operation, assisting at the operation and learning about post-operative care of the patient.

How could I be sure about my intense positive feelings for Victoria?

When I was alone in the evenings my thoughts were high-jacked with doubts. Did I really love her or was it that I was lonely and tired? I physically craved Victoria yet misgivings kept getting in the way, especially when I was fatigued. Was she my ideal mate, or was Mother right when she had blurted out that Victoria wasn't suitable for me? I was affronted by her statement and I resented her opinion for I felt she was categorically wrong. So, why was I having all these qualms? And, was Victoria having them too?

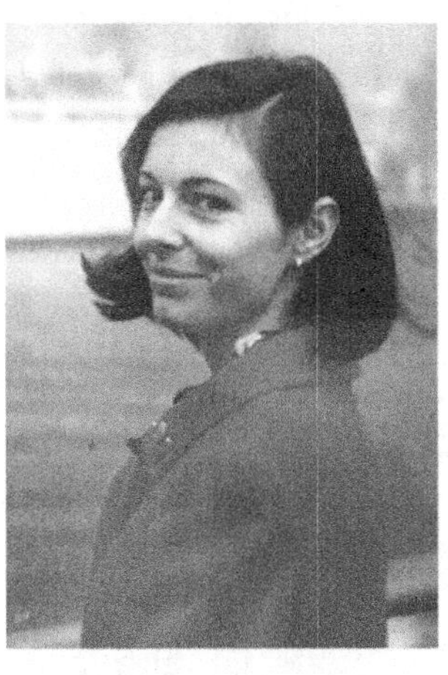

Was this the appropriate time for such a commitment when we were expecting to be all consumed by further training; I by surgery and Victoria by completing medical school and her specialty training in pediatrics? These activities would consume the next two years of our lives. During this period would we have the time to love and nurture each other? Would we have time to live life together in the fragments of time we could find?

Without her physical presence and with the draining feeling of distrust that existed since Mother abandoned me as a child, my uncertainty kept resurfacing. Trust was a fragile wound that kept reopening. I feared our bonds might weaken over time since we would be frequently apart during our training. This negative feeling was exacerbated by the chronic lack of sleep, the fatigue of the long hours at work and the thought that I was being neglected by her.

Despite feeling exhausted I sat down in Vanderbilt Hall and wrote Victoria an aerogram, pouring out my endless love and devotion to her.

> My dearest, sweetest, darling Victoria,
> God knows how much I miss you and how I love and cherish you. If living apart

from you is what I'd have to do to get a training here, I'd gladly forsake Harvard just to be close to you all the time. I miss your voice, your aura, your smell, your body, and think of you endlessly. I love you so much. Being alone makes me feel unwanted, unloved, and unfulfilled. I need you by my side, just to feel secure and complete.

The medical students at Harvard are a few years older than at UCH—of course! They go to a four-year liberal arts college before medical school. Unlike us, they seem to know exactly what they want to do in life AND where they are going to live in this huge country. I bask in the spirit of collegiality and camaraderie, overwhelmed by their spontaneous generosity and kindness. I tell them about you, how smart you are, how I adore you, and what a great doctor you'll be.

I love you so much. Adieu for now. See you in my dreams.

Love forever,
Your Marwan

Rising from my worktable and despite the late hour in the day, I went to mail the aerogram at the front desk. It was dark and cold outside. The clerk said my letter could take up to a week to reach London.

"A week?"

"Yeah," he said, shrugging his shoulders. "Could be less. But I'd count on a week or so."

The thought that my emotions would take that long to reach her and she wouldn't know in the meantime how I felt about her was torture. And the *very notion* that her reply would also take a week to reach me was agony. I might lose her during this time.

The anguish of the silence; the torment of my insecurity was brutalizing.

I decided to telephone. As I stood in Vanderbilt's phone booth armed with a handful of coins, a very sweet and young-sounding AT&T operator helped me reach Victoria on the Isle of Wight. We were overjoyed at hearing each other's voices—and so clearly. Her comforting voice soothed my demons of anxiety, insecurity and fear.

As she spoke, my brain was flooded with the memory of our sexual pheromones and the proximity of her warm body.

"My rotation ends two weeks early. Can you imagine that," I said, uncertain of her response. And whispering so that her mother didn't hear, I suggested, "We could spend a couple of weeks together in Antigua." Mindful of her proper background, I went on that perhaps it might be best if we first got married.

"Are you proposing?"

"Yes, yes."

She accepted immediately. I could hear her yelling the news to her mother, followed by hoots and cheers, presumably from Shirley and the others who were there. The offer excited Victoria. She whispered, "That's such good news. Now I won't have to worry about arranging a posh wedding that mummy envisages when she is manic and I know she'd not be up to managing." She ended by saying, "I love you so very much."

As we talked while I fed coins at the prompt of the operator, our plans developed and unfolded in the mania of love. We would marry in a registry office or at the British Consulate in Boston. We would have a Caribbean honeymoon at a time when only the British rich and famous, including royalty, scandalized those exotic isles as reported in the London Tabloids. Since my finals were looming in May of 1968, Victoria said she'd find us a flat near UCH and near several Tube stations affording access to Westminster Medical School, where Victoria was training.

I was elated. Victoria's first letter arrived. She had started writing it after I had departed. I could hear her voice while reading it—engulfed by her perfume.

> Darling,
> How are you my far away love? I miss you. Life has become a vague mixture of carrying on, which I feel apart from—if you see what I mean—I feel dissociated, as if part of me was elsewhere—i.e., is and was you. I love you. So many questions to ask you—so many things I didn't manage to, but wanted to say when you left due to my emotions—I don't think I even wished you *bon voyage*!

She concluded with,

> I love you forever and ever.

Intoxicated by her fragrance and script I kissed each word. In the dimness of my cold dorm room, her words were sublime—reassuring and assuaging my lonesomeness. I read and reread her letter seemingly a thousand times, dreaming that she was in my arms. I savored every word, seeing her writing it in my mind's eye and wanting to cling to her, kiss her, and love her.

After spending ten days almost continuously in the hospital, engrossed surgically, enjoying myself and living in my new world, my first free weekend loomed. To fill my time, I planned to catch up on sleep and study my surgical text and read the notes I had taken on diseases I had witnessed and their surgical treatment. Since I constantly had fresh "Kildare suits," I really had no laundry to do. Most evenings, I wrote to Victoria.

> My dearest wife to be,
> I love and miss you. Your voice was so clear as if it came from next door instead of the thousand kilometers across the Atlantic. It was so very clear that I wanted to crawl down the line and hold you in my arms. I have some additional news.
>
> Do you remember Prof. Huxley's secretary who had helped me with proofing the first issue of *Potential* and the issues that followed? She now works for the new head of physiology here. When she heard of our plans to marry in Boston, she had a whole group of students who are with me in surgery over for tea to celebrate!
>
> Funny really because no tea was served, only coffee, beer, and soft drinks. We sat about the floor. When I said that

you were coming Sunday, December 10 and that we would be getting married two or three days later before going to Antigua. They were pretty excited. Stu suggested that we could stay at his flat near Fenway Park, and Edith offered to give me a ride to Logan Airport to meet you.
Now here is the nasty news. Apparently, there is a prerequisite three-day residency in Massachusetts before we can marry.

And imagine this: a federal law that both partners have to have a negative Wassermann blood test for syphilis. My friends discussed potential solutions to solve our tight schedule. Please don't worry my love, I'll find an answer and share it with you in my next letter. I will overcome all barriers in my determination to make you mine.

Love always,
Marwan

On a separate sheet I listed my week's numerous operations and sent it along. I also mentioned my surprise that someone had intimated that years ago one of the surgeons who had come from UCH had a mistress while he was in Boston. I made it clear to her that would never be the case with me. Further, I added that I couldn't understand why someone thought this was a topic worth mentioning to me. Was it mere gossip, which as you know I hate? Such matters occurred in both Egypt and

Europe—every society, country and land. Victoria's next scented letter focused on this particular issue.

Darling
Your work sounds fascinating—hope it's not too hard on you. I'm glad you're having such fun, etc. How do you know that the English surgeon had a mistress while he was there? This is the thing I don't like about men. They assume if they're away from their wife for any length of time, they are expected to and thus do have a mistress—(this isn't a dig at you, my love—now—but I hope this won't have to ever happen in the future, altho' it would be partly my fault if it did).

I'm longing to come, but there's just so much to do I don't know where to begin—a flat, end-of-term exams next week, fun, drinks, party, Xmas pies, and keeping sane!! My darling, I will write tomorrow in less of a hurry. I love you and want you. All my love,

Your Vicki

A lipstick imprint of her lips ended the letter.

I kissed the imprint repeatedly and inhaled her perfume. Her reply stunned me and put me in a different mental state. Never mind who it was or if it was true or mere gossip? Did she assume all men behaved like her stereotype? Her assumption that a mistress would be *"partly my fault"* disturbed me. What did that mean? Was she projecting the sins of her father? I was perplexed, almost hurt that she would dwell on this aspect of an otherwise long letter to her.

Three letters arrived the following day—one from Victoria, one from Oma and one from Mother. Victoria had rapturous news: "Have I told you I found a small, cheery flat near the hospital? 15 Albany Street, Regent's Park, N.W.1. I hope we'll be happy there together my love." She had penned fourteen kisses —oh, how I wanted each one! I imagined them, our lips touching and getting progressively more passionate. I wondered if there would be some left over to hungrily plant on her naked body.

The second envelope was from Oma. I delighted in receiving notes from her. In keeping with her kind disposition, she wished Victoria and me a life of happiness together. The last one was from Mother. I opened it with trepidation. After all the negative vibes about my bride, I hoped it had an encouraging tone.

Sunday Night, November 26, 1967

Well, son, I had a long conversation with Vicky tonight when she informed me of the delightfully <u>small</u> flat she found at long last, suitably situated near Portland Place. I feel sure you both have a happy and satisfying life and careers before you. She is a sweet girl! . . . and you will be happy together–the best foundation for a true partnership.

I hear from Vicky that you are returning to UCH on 1 January. In this case, I

```
shall have my bunions cut off at the end
of January at UCH.
```

At least she wished us well, this time. Quite a shift from her previous attitude about Victoria and me. As was typical, her three-page typed letter mixed health, financial and family issues, with instructions for me to write to her friends in Cairo, Germany and England—friends "who took care of her affairs," for which she perceived she needed a man, her son, by her side. It ended with a lengthy diatribe about my sister Gulnar and her husband, Freimut, their distance from her, and their financial shenanigans. I folded up her letter, feeling quite exhausted, and reread Oma's and Victoria's letters for comfort.

The emotional tug to England was Victoria. If we came to work and study in the United States, how would she like or adapt to life here? How would we survive emotionally and physically when we would both expect to be the primary person in our union—-each in intense training situations? Who would be number one without subverting the other person's life?

4

PLANS, PLANS, PLANS

Time present and time past,
Are both perhaps present in time future,
And time future contained in time past.
—T. S. Eliot

A run of sunny days raised my spirits. Letters from Victoria arrived almost every other day, despite which I desperately missed her. This feeling of being unconnected was a source of apprehension. Apprehension of what exactly? Why the disquiet for my Victoria? I yearned for and missed our passion and intimacy; her letters were no substitute for closeness—they were passionless. Victoria peppered her letters with "I love you," and "I want you." Yet, with each note I wanted more. I wanted bolder words of permissive encouragement, emotional words, phrases that vividly expressed her erotic longing for me, for my body—words dripping with amorous tenderness, words that conjured and fired up my imagination with sexual wanting.

Words similar to those that Magdalena used to send me

during her last few days of longing for me when we were in Cairo and then in letters from Poland: "I want to feel the weight of your body on me," and "to hug your strong shoulders" and "to have my legs hold you." The imagery that her sweet words evoked left me in suspended wonder. Unfortunately, our relationship hadn't reached that stage. So, feeling less than clean, I'd flush the letters she'd sent to me in Manchester down the toilet and then I'd immediately expunged them from my memory feeling acutely embarrassed. I looked around. Had anyone seen me reading them?

Then, at sixteen, I was not as much in love with her as I was now with Victoria at twenty-three. Perhaps that was the difference between reserved British women and continental girls. Victoria was special. I had held her. I had explored. I had become intoxicated with her scent, her giggles, her warmth, and now the time to when she'd arrive seemed impossibly forever. A time I'd just have to survive.

In Victoria's next letter, she wrote the words I had wanted to hear: "Darling I so long to be with you—just to be in your arms + be warm and scrunched and lying near your warm, alive body, yummy!" In my heart, I truly felt that the genuine basis of my security was close physical contact with Victoria. Her giving, her touch, was my refuge.

I had seen the effect of touching an unconscious patient in the ICU. Their pulse, heart rate and breathing changed in response to the comfort of touch. The surgeon poet Spencer Michael Free had also expressed similar sentiments in his poem, "The Human Touch"—*the touch of the hand and the sound of the voice sing on in the soul always.* I ached for Victoria's unique touch, for when it came and lingered our heart rates certainly changed. It signaled reassurance, comfort, *I'm here for you.*

———

Through Professor Huxley's secretary, I learned that the surgical unit at UCH was in upheaval after Professor Pilcher had retired. This was followed by a slow exodus of younger surgical staff, some to other hospitals and others immigrating to South Africa and Canada. My plan to apply for the house surgeon's job seemed in jeopardy. Further, I suspected I did not stand a chance compared to a British candidate. Perhaps after marrying Victoria and getting the unique and prestigious BTA, I might be viewed differently by the British system—one of "our boys." Nevertheless, just like I had in Egypt, I had to develop a Plan B.

Americans embraced modernization in science, technology and medicine. I saw the transformative impact of medical innovation daily during my stay at Mass General—in the OR, ICU and ER. I witnessed their determination and drive for achievement and wanted to be part of that wave, to contribute to this environment. The little voice inside my head that said, "get your training here," progressively grew louder, becoming almost an obsession. As I understood it, one first became an intern on the general surgical service. If all went well one cycled up to become a first-year resident then a second-year resident and upwards to a fifth-year or chief resident—all the while being supervised by a fully trained attending or staff member. At each stage one received progressively more responsibility for the patient and acquired greater operative skill—skills imparted/taught by one's seniors, be they attendings or even senior residents. The advantage was that you became known to those who trained and supervised you.

The supervision and who taught or guided a researcher was less clear when one went into the laboratory and did bench research. Projects usually took two years to complete, allowing one's wife to work and one's children to attend the same school.

If I were to complete the five-year surgical residency program, it would be to my benefit when I returned home, for I could then apply to sit for both fellowships—the American and Royal colleges—the latter only if I did the Primary Fellowship.

After being a few weeks at Mass General I felt that in America, the training of young surgeons was much more rigorous and systematic relative to back home. I'd have to do two six-month rotations at different hospitals before I could sit for the Primary and if I was so lucky to be one of the twenty percent to passed it, I'd look for a two-to-four-year Registrar/Residency hopefully with some supervision. Only after that could I sit for the final Fellowship exam in Britain. Then I'd have to look for a Senior Registrar position before finding a Consultancy job within the National Health Service. And throughout, we'd be living in different towns and hopefully Victoria would also have a job in the same geographical vicinity. In the U.S., I would train in one town and when I had finished I could hang-up my shingle and start operating independently. What a huge difference.

I asked Dr. Sugarbaker how I would set about applying for residency. "Since you are interested in research perhaps a better fit for you is the Peter Bent Brigham—the other Harvard training hospital chaired by the dynamic Dr. Francis D. Moore."

"Oh!"

"The Brigham is near Vanderbilt Hall, behind the medical school building. Since it's now resident selection time, you should make an appointment to see him right away."

I telephoned Dr. Moore's office, and his secretary gave me an appointment in two weeks—the day after Victoria would arrive. I would have to mention this in my next letter to her. Fancy pursuing potential surgical jobs after she arrived, I thought, when we hadn't even enough time to get reacquainted, to know each other after a six-week absence! Six weeks that felt like an eternal delay of our love—emotional and physical. Like holding my breath for six weeks and gasping for love when she was in my arms. And, she'd be jet lagged.

"If you are serious," Tom chimed in, "You really need to apply to at least a dozen programs. Getting into a top-notch surgical residency is highly competitive." I was alarmed at the prospect of applying so late in the selection season. Was I wasting my time trying to compete with local talent?

Stu brought a green tome that listed all the residencies in the United States. I plowed through the book and concluded I would focus on Boston or New York, which were closer to England. I arranged two interviews in New York on December 14, Victoria's twenty-third birthday. That day we'd be in New York and in the evening fly to Antigua for our real honeymoon —sea, sand and sex.

I shared with Victoria my thoughts and tentative plans that we should perhaps both train in Boston or New York. To soften the blow, I mentioned the upheaval at UCH following Professor Pilcher's retirement. Apparently, the new professor was from Leeds. He had brought with him his own staff. As an unknown, I thought I stood no chance of getting a position as house surgeon on the unit. These developments might make her more sympathetic to my career concerns although I worried that interviews were hardly post-wedding activities.

Arrangements were falling into place. Victoria was her usual efficient, dependable self and had managed to get a lot done—travel arrangements, clothes shopping with Shirley, finding a small love nest in Albany Street and passing her numerous end-of-term exams. She was to arrive on Sunday, December 10. I longed to kiss every precious inch of her body. With all these arrangements in place, I could focus on preparing for my upcoming oral exam.

Drs. Rodkey of the White Service and Wang of the Ward Service were my examiners for the thirty-minute oral test. Waiting in my suit and tie outside the room before being called, my hands were sweating. I rationalized that if I did not do well, no one would really care and I could return to London.

Dr. Rodkey was a young man with a shock of dark hair who was prone to break easily into a smile, endearing him to the residents, myself included. I had assisted him on a couple of cases on the private service and enjoyed his commonsense approach toward surgical problems. Dr. Wang was one of the more established surgeons and was experienced in abdominal diseases. He gave several lectures to students and taught using the Socratic method. They made me feel at ease by being very complimentary about my contributions on the surgical service and asking how I had enjoyed myself in Boston. Even so, I remained on guard, not sure how the exam was going to proceed.

Dr. Wang asked how I would manage a patient with Crohn's disease—chronic inflammatory bowel disease that affects the lining of the digestive tract—who was admitted with bleeding. I answered succinctly, having attended his lecture. Dr. Grant asked the next question: How I would manage an elderly patient in the ER with an incarcerated hernia? Once more I was able to answer appropriately. They alternated, asking me progressively more challenging questions, probing the boundaries of my knowledge. When the questions became too complicated and beyond my knowledge, I heard myself say, "I am not certain how to manage such a patient but I know how to look it up."

They seemed pleased with the answer and concluded the exam by asking me when I would be returning to London. I took the opportunity to mention that my fiancée was arriving and that I planned a couple of residency interviews before we went on our honeymoon. The allotted time for the oral test flew by, and it was over all too soon. I exited the exam room feeling I had done well enough and was pleased with myself. I shared my feeling of euphoria in an aerogram mailed to London.

As Victoria's arrival time approached, the one problem I had not yet resolved was paying for a Wassermann test for syphilis required by Massachusetts prior to marriage. My fellow students suggested I donate a unit of blood, for which the hospital would pay me $50. I would use that to pay for our tests. My colleagues felt sure that prior to my blood donation, they routinely check the donor's blood for syphilis, permitting the chief of the blood bank, a surgeon, to attest to my negative status. Perhaps I could persuade him, given the mitigating circumstances, to sign the form stating that Victoria, too, was syphilis free.

When the laboratory chief, also a surgeon, discovered I was from UCH he was overjoyed. Reminisces poured out about his time at the National Institute for Medical Research in London as a research fellow while a technician drew my blood.

"Tell me about your bride. Was she previously married?"

"No," I said, somewhat surprised.

He proceeded to cross-examine me concerning Victoria's background.

"She is a medical student who comes from a proper and conservative upper-class British family on the Isle of Wight," I said.

"I used to go sailing down there. Great fun."

"In fact, when I met her," I hesitated, looking straight into his eyes before continuing almost in a whisper, "I think she was a virgin." Raising my voice, I added, "You will enjoy meeting her, for she is arriving next Sunday, December 10."

He nodded sympathetically. Producing a form, he signed, attesting that she, too, was syphilis free. "As soon as she lands on Sunday, repeat Sunday, she comes to the blood bank to have her blood drawn. Come back on Monday morning to collect both your forms."

I felt special. That's what I would have done. We were in the same profession and as the saying goes, "There is honor among . . ." in this case, physicians. The requirements of residency in Massachusetts and a negative syphilis test were indeed quaint and did not exist in England.

I telephoned Victoria to share the good news. Hearing her voice was heavenly. It transported me to a place of reverie. There was truth to the proverb that absence makes the heart grow fonder. It certainly did.

Victoria's last letter arrived on Saturday, December 9, 1967—she was primed like a rocket on a launch pad ready to blast off . . . trajectory aimed at BOSTON, destination ME! Her landing site . . . MY ARMS.

How could I wait?

5

THE BINDING OF BONDS

I have spread my couch
With dyed Egyptian linen,
Sprinkled my bed
With myrrh, aloes, and cinnamon.
Come, let us drink our fill of love,
Let us make love all night long!
Book of Proverbs 7: (16-18)

The rumor swirling that a wildcat strike by BOAC staff had grounded some flights added an air of uncertainty to the waiting crowd expecting passengers. Was my Victoria's flight affected? Cancelled?

Those gathering became restless as time passed and we lived in uncertainty. Edith and I stood about wondering who could give us an accurate status report, when an announcement declared the arrival of her flight. It was only an hour late. Victoria and my separation was about to be over.

Edith remained with me as we waited impatiently outside the Logan arrivals. A solid door to the immigration hall separated the "Land of the Free" from the rest of the world beyond. Whenever it opened, dazed travelers stepped out, looked around until a smile crossed their jet-lagged faces, and they rushed forward into the embraces awaiting them.

When, finally, Victoria came through our eyes met instantly in blazing happiness. She looked stunning. Edith gasped at the ravishing vision.

Victoria wore her mother's mink coat, which flapped open over a red dress and slender legs in tall high heels. When she saw Edith by my side, she froze and the joy on her face turned into a mystified frown. I had barely introduced her to Edith when Victoria asked, "Do you still love me?" There was no kiss, not even a cheek kiss, and certainly no embrace. Only a heavy air of suspicion. What had prompted this? Astonished, I explained that, compared to London, public transport in Boston was rudimentary and that Edith, *a fellow student*, as I emphasized had kindly volunteered to drive us to the apartment as I had mentioned in my letter.

I felt terrible. Was I going to have to earn her love every day? Why? Was she always going to make me feel guilty every time I was with a female colleague? Did she not trust her own power of attractiveness and my undying love for her?

Her emotional coldness evoked painful yet ever-present memories, like a skin rash that never went away, of my wanting to be wanted. Was this how our relationship would evolve? The same coldness and distancing I put up with from Mother? The very thought dampened my mood. All the anticipation, all the pent-up love fizzled out of me. I could see she too was less exuberant than I had expected her to be—than her letters had portrayed or I had foolishly built up. Just because I was practical enough to accept a fellow student's offer for a ride? If I wasn't cash strapped then I should have taken a taxi. I wondered whether Victoria was living with the fear of her father's double life and projecting it on me.

Edith drove us through Boston's heavy traffic to Mass General in silence, parked her car and waited. Victoria and I ascended to the blood bank, and even a peck on her cheek didn't change her bearing. What was her problem? Where was her enthusiasm for me? Maybe it was just jet lag.

Victoria had her blood drawn. She was familiar with the agreement I had reached with chief of the blood bank. We descended in silence. She must be tired.

Edith kindly drove us up Massachusetts Avenue, direction Fenway, to Stu's apartment. Victoria got out while I profusely, yet embarrassedly, thanked Edith, who, as a budding psychiatrist, sensed the tension. To lighten the mood, I expressed to Victoria my curiosity at Stu's naked female mannequin who greeted us in the dark and dingy hall. I had never seen such an imaginative sexy garment. My fiancée did not share my delight, frowning at my eagerness to examine them and to engage in my speculation about where I could get her something similar.

I attributed her lack of interest in me and the novel unique situation to jet lag, fatigue, to the cultural shock, and to what appeared to be the beginnings of an upset stomach. The poor girl wasn't feeling well. She went to bed feeling unwell and tired from the stress of travel. She was also probably dehydrated. What could I do to help her? By nature I was a problem solver, yet I felt helpless and was hoping a good night's sleep and a meal would revive her.

I was so thrilled to have her with me at last—merely in the same room breathing the same air. Overjoyed, I wanted to embrace her, to hold her, to hear her stories of the last six weeks and share my exciting experiences in Boston before eagerly sliding into bed. But she had already fallen asleep—a pang of sympathy overcame me. She must have had several weeks of busy anxiety leading to this moment. Who wouldn't have, after all? I was expecting too much of her. Even in slumber she looked divine and exquisitely beautiful—my darling Victoria.

Jet lag roused her early and I awoke excited at the anticipated day's events as we breakfasted at McDonald's—a novel experience for both of us. I wanted to hear all about our flat, her mother, anything just to hear her voice. I could not keep my eyes off her—her vivid smile showed her dimples and white teeth, and her eyes were dancing. She wore the red suit over a colorful blouse and had a string of pearls. Her freshly cut hair was shoulder length, and she had swept it behind her ears, exposing the pearl earrings I had bought her on our trip to Wedel a couple of years ago when I wanted to introduce Victoria to my real mother—Oma. "*Sie ist doch schön . . .*" Oma had said adding, "*Ja gantz net.*" My grandmother thoroughly approved of my choice. Not so important was Gulnar's ratification of my wife to be—my bar of expectation was low for I didn't expect anything from her.

Victoria had recovered her rosy, loving self. I stretched my hand out across the table grasping hers. It was warm and soft, so soft I wanted to kiss her palm and run my tongue across it. Looking into her eyes did not prevent me from looking longingly at her lily-white cleavage. She had tracked my gaze and acknowledged my intent. She read me and my desires with a smile. I wanted to take her off to bed, to hold her and collect all the kisses and hundreds of "I love yous" I had read in her letters that I had only been able to dream about.

We were re-familiarizing ourself with each other; we needed privacy and a congenial environment—other than McDonald's.

We walked across Government Center arm in arm toward the Charles heading to Mass General to collect our blood syphilis certificates. Even though it was an early Monday morning, we encountered few people. It didn't matter. There could have been a crowd. All I felt was that we were one, alone strolling with design in lockstep, Victoria clung to my left arm, shoulder to my side, hip to hip, and gazed happily at me, I at her, occasionally watching out where we stepped. Her eyes were their sparking self and spoke of infinite contentment. Yes, I was the luckiest man in Boston . . . no, in the world. My Victoria was at long last by my side glittering in the morning sun, smiling joyfully—I felt like a man, a man with the fantastic woman who completed his life. One unit of ecstasy, a man intoxicated with rarefied Mass General air and a surgical future, a man striving for everything of which he dreamt, a man full of exhilaration. Above all one with confidence. She, too, must have had that feeling of being with a man she could count on, a man she could lean on, a man who wanted her to fulfill her dreams. These two sets of feelings formed a single unit, the Meguid wholeness.

At the blood bank the technicians were busy—the chief had not arrived. Our certificates vouched us to be syphilis free, and with no one person to thank in particular for their diligence in facilitating the next step toward our union, we left, Victoria's mink coat turning several heads on the way. I never doubted Victoria's Wasserman test would be negative, and we joked, thinking of Shirley's wicked wit: "Only Bishops and liars get syphilis off toilet seats!"

We ambled back across Government Center hand in hand in the bright sunlight of that crisp December morning to the Municipal Courthouse. Maybe the crisp, biting fresh air and the piercing sunrays added to Victoria feeling even better. She had brought the white gold wedding ring with her, which she had slipped into my suit pocket before we left Stu's condo.

I had bought it from Mrs. Goldberg's antique jewelry shop in Woburn Place, London, in August, almost a year after getting the engagement ring, at a time when Victoria and I first talked about a potential marriage date. I tried to keep the purchase a secret because I was very excited. Mrs. Goldberg badgered me repeatedly, saying that it might need sizing, more I think in the aim of getting Victoria into her jewelry shop to sell another item. I resisted. Had she forgotten that I was a mere student on a tight budget?

I finally gave in and showed it to Victoria with a great sense of pride when we were alone. The moment she slipped it on, I felt an extra surge of love and abiding affection. It fit perfectly. Right away! And with it on her finger, I knew I had snagged this precious woman—my life's partner. She took it off and kept it safe until, as she whispered to me, "the real moment." The emotions of just talking about *that* moment had led to passionate lovemaking.

We had an eleven o'clock meeting with Peter Wright, my fellow UCH medical student. He turned out to be the other person with whom I shared my room at Vanderbilt, although one wouldn't know it because he never slept there the nights I was in nor even the weekends. I came across him from time to time in the cafeteria. He wasn't an effusive character and was uncomfortable with eye contact. He agreed to be our best man and witness the marriage.

"When?"

"Tuesday December 12th. at the Registration office in the Government Center."

"I'll miss the beginning of a lecture, so don't be late."

"Don't you want to join us in a festive lunch?"

"Oh, no. I'll run back as soon as its over to get to the noon-time lecture. It's in the Ether Dome. It'll be crowded. You don't want to miss it," he added. And just before he turned away and disappeared, he repeated, "You won't be late, will you?"

"No. Don't worry."

Justice of the Peace, Emile N. Winkler, performed the ceremony, if that is what one could call it, for it was very brief. There was no family, no well-wishing friends, not even strangers hanging around. Only the two of us standing in front of the Justice and Peter hanging around in the background.

I do not remember what we vowed, if anything, only that I was in ecstasy standing next to Victoria on the threshold of our life together.

When requested, I fumbled about in my pocket to find the band and slipped it on her finger. It complemented her white platinum engagement ring. This *was* the "the real moment." When told to kiss the bride, to my surprise she presented her cheek. I delivered a peck. On our way out, I paid $5 and Peter, our witness, signed our wedding certificate and hurried off having constantly glanced at his watch throughout the fifteen-minute proceedings.

No bells rang and no angels sang. Our marriage in Boston was a formality. No one objected to our union, no others joined us to make it festive and joyous. Victoria was beginning to feel unwell, and I was still in a mental state—working mode. Why hadn't I invited my fellow classmates—I, foolishly, had not planned. I had not appreciated what a momentous occasion this was for a woman and for a man. I had no defense other than the limited supply of greenbacks.

This was the antithesis of a fancy ostentatious wedding on the Isle of Wight. In our forty-two years of our union, I always regretted getting married this way. Shirley's way, with flowers, music, with Uncle John walking Victoria down the aisle and giving her away, with tears and cheers in some little country church followed by a second honey-moon, would have been exquisite. We should have eloped to the Caribbean just to be together, but the old-fashioned conservative me chose propriety over adventure and audaciousness—just as paltry as my parents' marriage in Marylebone, London in 1939.

But in 1967 Boston, Victoria smiled and put her arm into

mine and we marched off in silence, looking for a restaurant. It was an inner joy to be finally wedded and I could not help sharing the news with our server at Warmuth's restaurant in Devonshire Street, who presented us with a teaspoon as a memento, our only material wedding present that day. And thinking back, I probably hadn't tipped adequately by American standards, or consistent with the presence of a gorgeous woman wearing a Mink coat.

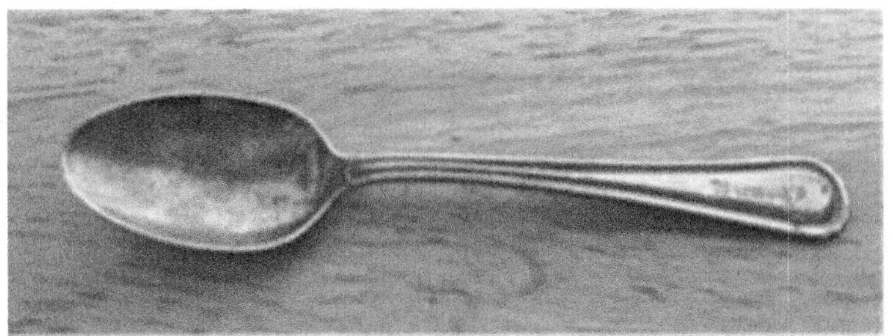

We sat alone at a table outside in December's midday sun, enjoying lobster with drawn butter and a baked potato, followed by an enormous helping of American ice cream.

Poor Victoria. She was beginning to fade fast, afflicted by jet lag for it must have been early evening in London. Worse, the heavy midday meal irritated her stomach bug—or was it an early winter flu as I was beginning to suspect? She could not eat much and wanted to return to Stu's apartment. Despite the important occasion in our life I had given little thought to planning our marriage for we were alone. It seemed hardly a festive event and I was sorry that neither members of Victoria's nor my family were with us to rejoice and share our happiness. Perhaps we could make amends when planning our celebration in London, after finals.

I was high on my surgical service experience, on the exam outcome, and on having Victoria with me. I wanted to attend the two o'clock lecture about cryopreservation of blood and to thank the blood bank chief. Above all I wanted to show off my beautiful new wife in her mink. I selfishly persuaded her, over her mild objections, to attend the lecture not fully realizing that she was really unwell. After all, was she not going to be a physician soon? She sat with her head on her folded arms on the desk in front of her, unable to focus, sacrificing for me. How very foolish of me.

The following morning, we sat outside Professor Francis D. Moore's office. Victoria felt somewhat better and accompanied me after I shared with her the disastrous news of the dissolution of the department of surgery at UCH and my Plan B. She looked glamorous. Hardly the paragon of a medical student.

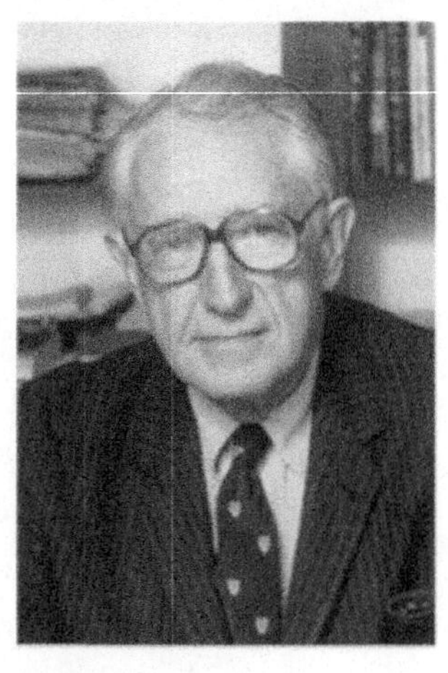

Dr. Moore opened the door, looking scholarly with his horn-rimmed glasses and graying temples. We stood and as we exchanged greetings his focus was on the young red-suited beauty with a mink. I introduced Victoria, who looked magnificent in her glamorous attire as she smiled and extended her hand. I mentioned that she had joined me from London a couple of days ago and that we married, "In Boston only yesterday."

"Yesterday? Well congratulations!" he said in a booming voice, oozing charm from every pore. This eminent surgeon impressed me. Victoria impressed him.

She remained outside for the interview. In his office, he fired off a series of questions—who was my father, what had he done, what did I want to do in life, and what were my research interests. For his last question he asked me the names of individuals I had worked with while on the White surgical service. The interview was over in ten minutes, in what I felt had been a mere formality.

Riding back on the bone-rattling T, I told Victoria, "That was a waste of time. He said he would write to me in London if he had a position available."

There was no comment. She didn't feel well.

Victoria took to bed. It must have been awful—a stomach virus, loose bowels and getting dragged around. I was becoming alarmed. She was increasingly manifesting more symptoms of a viral infection: rapid fatigue, upset stomach, bowel irritation, and maybe even a fever. She rolled up into a ball and went to sleep. I worried. If matters got worse, who would I call? Was there a GP? What meds could I give her and where would I buy them? I fretted. What if she didn't get better?

After an afternoon nap I was relieved to see Victoria was feeling better. We took a taxi to Professor Huxley's secretary's flat where my friends had planned a gathering to welcome Victoria and celebrate our union. We sat crossed-legged on the floor. Victoria unwrapped a small wedding present. A Snoopy card contained a silver JFK coin.

Victoria and I had been together for forty-eight hours and married, yet there had not been a tender moment between us. We had not shared all those kisses and longing moments so passionately penned in her twenty-two letters. The emotions seemed so difficult to express in person, reminding me of Jane Austen's comment: *If I loved you less, I might be able to talk about it more.* I felt that there was a space between us, one I could not fathom—like a cushion of solid air keeping us apart, as if we were strangers and had never shared moments of intimacy before. Was this the effect of six week's separation? Illness?

Poor planning on my part? Or, too great an expectation given the circumstances in play?

In our usual London medical environment, we had clung to each other—inseparable. Did we really know each other outside of that environment? We had never been alone or just by ourselves for any length of time. I hoped that she would feel better once she had slept it off and we could resume being our normal selves again.

Professor Moore sent a letter to London. We were in Antigua. The letter went to the hospital, where it lay around for several months, unattended and unanswered.

HARVARD MEDICAL SCHOOL
DEPARTMENT OF SURGERY

FRANCIS D. MOORE, M.D.
Moseley Professor of Surgery

Peter Bent Brigham Hospital
721 Huntington Avenue
Boston, Massachusetts 02115
Telephone 617 - 566-6226

December 15, 1967

Mr. Marwan MeGuid
University College Hospital
London
England

Dear Marwan:

Merely a note to set down on paper the fruits of our discussion of recent date.

We frequently appoint three to five Junior Assistant Residents above the level of Intern, who have not interned here with us.

You would be a candidate for such a position, and we would be quite interested in making such an offer to you.

However, we must settle up about these things no later than the 15th of October, 1968. I gave you a November date, and I think I was a little tardy on that. We should hear from you in October.

At that time, we can communicate with some of the surgeons with whom you have been working at University College Hospital, and then firm up an appointment for July 1, 1969.

Such an appointment would be in the regular mainstream of our clinical work, but it would also give you an opportunity in the laboratory if you so wished.

Good luck, and all best wishes in your forthcoming marriage!

And I will look forward to hearing from you next year.

Very truly yours,

Francis D. Moore, M.D.

FDM:kh

6

ANTIGUA HONEYMOON

Honeymoons are the beginning of wisdom but the beginning of wisdom is the end of romance.
—Helen Rowland

I had scheduled two interviews in New York, so after our breakfast on the flight from Boston, we went to Columbia, where the setting and presentation by the head of the residency program were so dismal that we rose and left during the presentation to the amazement of the other applicants. "You're just going to walk out? Wow. This is one of the finest surgical residencies," one whispered to me as I rose to leave. Little did I know that one day members of this fine institute would save my life. The quirks of fate!

We headed to our noontime interview at Roosevelt Hospital. When the senior surgeon who was to interview me met Victoria and discovered that it was her birthday, he graciously invited us to lunch in a nearby fancy restaurant. He spoke alluringly about life in New York—its art galleries and musical venues. While discussing the merits of Roosevelt's surgical residency he included Victoria, promising her an opportunity to train in pediatrics.

We parted having spent a good three pleasant and congenial hours together. Both Victoria and I had the impression that working at Roosevelt Hospital might be an agreeable opportunity.

Finally, we were on our way to Antigua. After six weeks of constant work and tension, my stress level ebbed. And, the virus found me—a stress-weakened, immune compromised host. Suddenly every bone in my body ached. After checking into the Antigua Beach Hotel, I fell into bed, physically and mentally exhausted. I felt as if I was going to die. Drifting between bouts of intense drowsiness and semiconsciousness, I kept repeating to my wife, "If I get worse take me to the American Hospital on the Island," repeating " . . . the *American* Hospital."

"Now you know how I felt in Boston," was her retort. I heard her and sympathized. Luckily, twenty-four hours later I was over the worst.

The glorious name "The Antigua Beach Hotel" was an oxymoron because it was nowhere near a beach. The American meal plan we signed up for provided only continental breakfast —fruit and cornflakes. We didn't have sufficient funds for a cooked breakfast, nor for lunch and dinner every day. Plus, the hotel was in a desolate part of the island—far from the beach and St. John's, the major town and capital.

We discussed our options and came up with some alternatives. I suggested a nifty idea. Why did we not introduce ourselves to the local medical community, starting with the hotel doctor, and offer our free services in exchange for hospitality? It worked—somewhat. The local GP, Dr. White, an elderly and portly Antiguan, introduced me to the young surgeon on the island.

I did rounds at the local eight-bed hospital with him,

Victoria in tow. Among the patients that we saw were two each with liver abscesses—conditions we did not see in London. He had drained each and mentioned that patient A was on one antibiotic and patient B was on a different one. I was impressed. "Are you doing a randomized study?"

"No man. Patients get whatever antibiotics we receive that day from the Red Cross." He then took me over to a chest half full of meds. I was taken aback. Here in the Caribbean, public hospitals were starving for adequate drugs. He showed me a state-of-the-art X-ray machine donated by the Canadian government. Sadly, it stood in the corner unplugged for lack of a technician. That night we had a splendid home-cooked Antiguan dinner in a congenial family environment. He would introduce us to an Austrian psychiatrist who ran the "Asylum" in St. John's saying he thought they had a room with two beds that we could occupy.

"And the beach?"

He shrugged his shoulders. "I don't have time for that. It's here for the tourists. St. John's," he added, "also has a tiny Barclay's bank and an equally small BOAC office along High Street. Both might become handy."

My other idea was not as practical. We took a taxi to the farmer's market and bought a stick of green bananas. We learned that they ripened from the bottom upward; with a bunch of seventy-two bananas, we would each have to eat six per day to keep up with their rate of ripening. We managed to avoid an expensive dinner that night, gorging on bananas. The next day for breakfast we had papaya, tea and cornflakes with condensed milk. I joyfully nicknamed it our honeymoon lunch/dinner plan.

We headed to the deserted beach. It was the right move, for the yellow sand, the waving palm trees, and the turquoise sea put us in the right mood to think we could finally start our honeymoon. We spread our towel on the sand and relaxed in the sun, which thawed our inhibitions as I lathered our bodies with suntan lotion and heard her gentle moans. I looked around for some privacy. Making love among the dunes was a common theme in the movies. Did the Antiguan's encourage this? Touching Victoria's skin had to suffice for now although we both wanted more.

Given my genes, my dark stripes, I browned very easily without burning. When we had baked sufficiently, we ran into a calm, cool sea, for there were no waves that day.

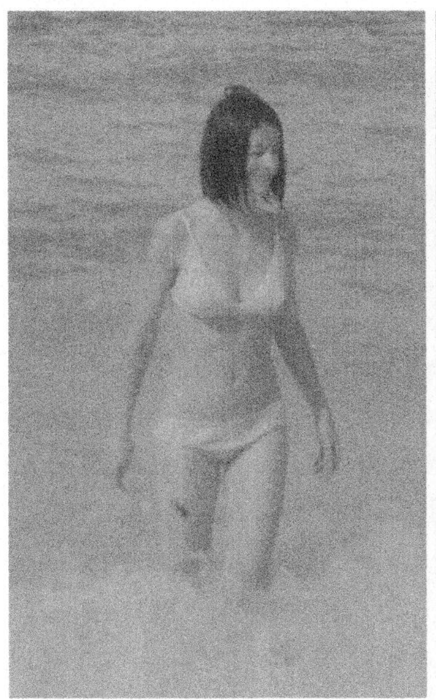

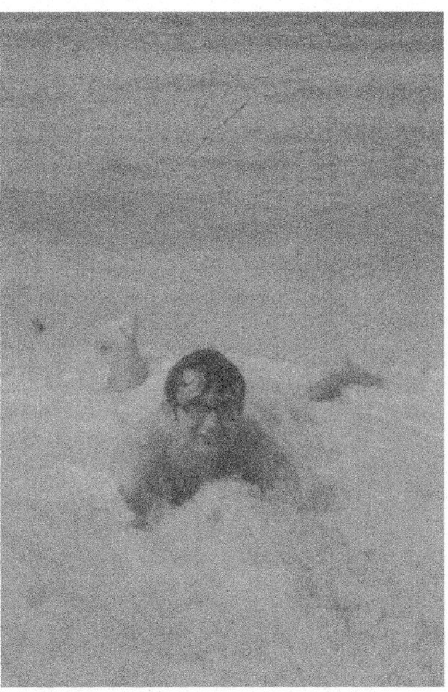

I found it refreshing, but for Victoria the water was too cold. We walked hand in hand along the beach. We were married now and this was our time together, time we had dreamed of and deserved—time to focus on each other and lavish affection. There was no outside world to intrude—no exams, no deadlines.

As we walked along with our feet in the warm Caribbean, an isolated figure appeared flickering in the hazy distance. The nebulous shimmer took on the form of a young man as he became more distinct. Surprised, I recognized him as a medical student from London. John had been a crewmember on the St. Bart's rowing team, which our University of London team had beaten in a race while rowing on the Thames a few years previously. As we drew abreast, he recognized me. The three of us stopped and introduced ourselves. "What a small world. What are you doing in Antigua?" I asked.

"I am a white Antiguan," he told us. "I live here. I'm visiting my parents before leaving tomorrow to spend Christmas in New York."

"How wonderful. You are lucky living here. We are on our honeymoon. Just got married. Poor as church mice." And I told him of our dilemma.

"My Aunt Maybelline and her retired husband, Delmar Drew, run a boarding house for retired army personnel at Half Moon Bay." He described the wide veranda surrounding the house, set in dense vegetation that sloped down to the pristine beach—a sturdy bungalow that had weathered many hurricanes. It was located on the leeward side of the island, some distance from St. John's. "I'll ask her if she can help you."

Hallelujah! What a coincidence. Could this potentially be our salvation?

Maybelline Drew was rotund, full of energy and empathy. "Of course, I can find room for two young honeymooners, even though they are as poor as church mice and have a huge banana stick," she drawled along in her delightful sing-song Caribbean English. "You know, if you eat too many of them and lie in the sun you will develop a rash," she felt obliged to tell us. "And do call me Mable."

It was a boarding house for single males—all ex-army, of different ranks and from different regiments. We moved into an empty room which had all we needed—a double bed, a shower and a flush toilet. For a modest price, we had a full English breakfast—two eggs, bacon and fried tomatoes with tea, toast and marmalade. For lunch, we reverted to eating our share of ripening bananas, although Victoria caught me out not eating my share.

Few of the guests availed themselves of tea—my favorite daily meal after breakfast. There were finger sandwiches, freshly baked scones with homemade strawberry jam, local honey and tea, of course. There was an honor-code bar for those who drank. "Which is what all these old army chaps do, starting much too early in the day, if you ask me," Mabel confided. She added, "I'll find you your own table since my guests are year-round residents and like to sit by themselves at their own table while nursing a drink. Dinner is served seven-thirty and I expect you to dress appropriately."

Our honeymoon began in earnest as we settled down for our afternoon siesta, together. That evening, as we stood in our finest, Victoria in her red suit, I in my gray one, both made for winter wear, Mabel introduced us to the patrons in the fully occupied dining room. She had arranged a small table for us. When she came to the part about our being on our honeymoon, there was much tittering and throat clearing among the elderly males—Colonels, Majors, and a variety of other ranks. Victoria was the sole female guest and her beauty radiated throughout the room. I viewed them as kindly "dirty old men." We were the odd happy couple and no doubt the source of their old memories and lewd fantasies.

A short path cut through the vegetation that led down to an immaculate beach. Delmar had placed some chairs and two chaise lounges on which we spread our towels and lay digesting our breakfast under coconut palms.

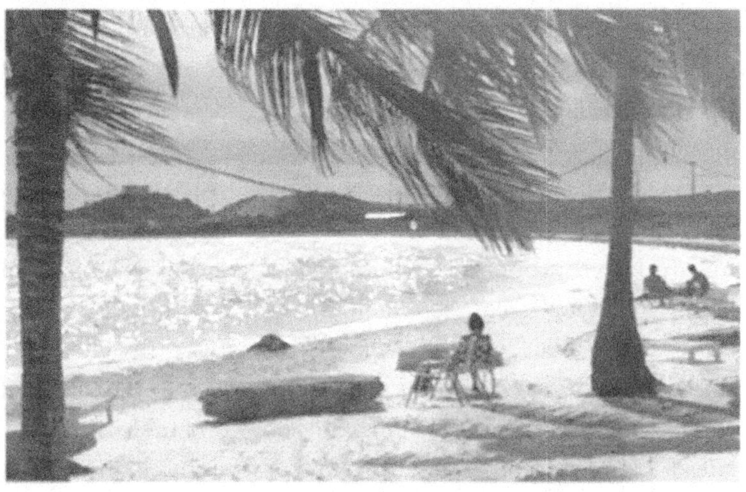

Despite the shade I browned in accordance to some of my genes while Victoria got a severe and nasty sunburn that made her sick once more. Victoria's fair complexion became lobster red—everywhere except where her skimpy bikini covered her. Her skin blistered, what we call severe first-degree skin burn. I could not touch her for a couple of days for fear of the pain although her breasts and where her skimpy bikini protected her remained lily-white. Rubbing soothing cream that Mable gave us on her shoulders, belly, legs and back was accompanied with cries of "Oh . . ." and "Ouches." Even the shower elicited pain.

My poor Victoria was in agony for two days. I felt bad for her. Light headed and nauseated. I pushed fluids and juices. I had no pain meds, not even aspirin—a mistake I'd never make again on my many future travels. First jet-lag, then a stomach bug, now a severe sunburn. So much for a honeymoon.

And for these couple of days her skin and body were off limits even as she lay naked on towels next to me. At such times a double bed was just too small for two persons. We spent two days indoors—lying in bed, dozing and reading. She carefully dressed for dinner.

As she improved, we agreed that the best way to get a tan was to expose ourselves to the sun's rays between 9 and 11 a.m. and then toast ourselves again, after our nap, between 4 and 6 p.m.

The Antiguan medical community, in a well-timed invitation, for we were both back to form, did not forget us. We were to visit the asylum. Delmar drove us to St. John's on one of his daily market runs. At the asylum we met the chief psychiatrist—an elderly physician who had escaped Austria believing he and his wife were on their way to America when the boat deposited him and several other Jewish families in the Caribbean. When our host discovered I was half German, he left us alone among the patients.

We wandered through the compound followed by a group of inmates who hailed us wildly as they trailed us, believing we were the King and Queen. Perhaps they knew my bride's name was Victoria. As far as I could tell, they suffered from florid schizophrenia. What were the chances that they were on expensive medications, when the surgical patients were making do with donated antibiotics? When I turned about to greet them with the hope of chatting with them, they scattered.

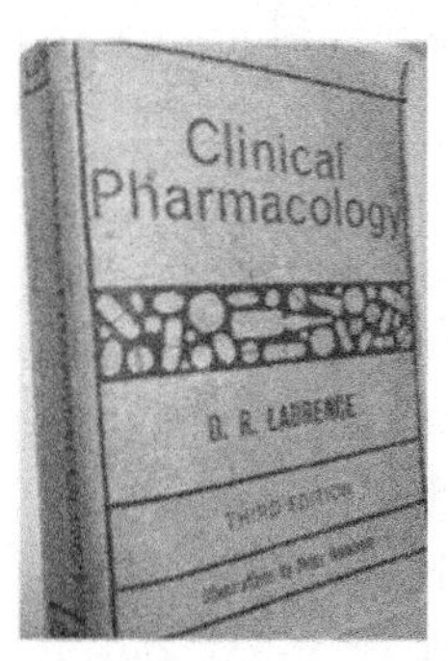

With the worst of the sun's injury over, we ventured back onto the beach. Victoria dozed and read her novel while I produced D.R. Laurence's *Clinical Pharmacology* textbook, knowing I had an exam soon after our return to London. In contrast to the pharmacology professor at University College, Professor Laurence—a clinical pharmacologist—was a dynamic lecturer. I had written a set of reasonably good notes and his book was humorously written and illustrated. Between lavishing my love on Victoria, lustily but gently rubbing her skin with heavy layers of sunscreen, admiring her good-looking bikini figure, cooling off in the Caribbean and our meals, I studied Laurence's text.

We rode once more with Delmar to St. John's when he was sent off to the market for produce needed for that evening's dinner. Beyond the asylum's gate on High Street, we found a Barclay's Bank with its inconspicuous entrance hidden among stalls of the local market that spilled onto the pavement. The entrance was narrow. The inside was also narrow with wooden floors and counters with iron bars separating us from the teller —relics from a past era.

Victoria produced her card and drew her daily allowance of £2. We did this several times during our stay, riding in with Delmar, drawing money, and riding back with him. We handed pounds sterling over to Mabel, who accepted them gladly in lieu of the local currency—the BIWI Dollar. We were unaware of the official conversion rate, which was seldom used—the dollar being used interchangeably by those who could.

The daily routine we established was relaxing. Lying on the beach reading Laurence, Victoria and I enjoyed the sun, the warm sand, and a quick dip in the cooling sea. I felt at one with my wife, I needed her, I wanted her, and now that I had her and she was mine to focus on, I put my concerns behind me—we seemed well suited.

Christmas Day was approaching. Mabel was busy preparing a special holiday feast. Delmar made numerous runs to the St. John's market, bringing back produce that his wife and her local helpers prepared. There would be one long table, covered with white linen, her best China, and wine glasses.

It was sweltering in the dining room on Christmas, despite the open windows and the slowly whirring ceiling fans. Outside, the sun shone brightly, making the room feel dim. The army of retired men wore their dress uniforms, all dripping with medals. We all quietly envied the one who wore the kilt.

We gorged on a full Christmas lunch interspersed with numerous raised glasses: "To the Queen." Given the full complement of inmates about the table, greater attention was paid to the food and drink than to making small talk. My attempt to chat to my neighbor who was hard of hearing or the Major with a bulbous, ruddy nose and prominent pores who sat opposite us was a dismal failure. They knew a WOG when they saw one. Besides, Victoria was much more interesting to admire and smile at in their illusory inebriation, even with a mouth full of turkey and sweet potatoes. Finally, someone rose and toasted, "The hostess, Mabel" for a topnotch dinner befitting the occasion. With a lot of chair scraping and "steady-as-we-go" comments, the intoxicates all stood, wabbled and steadied themselves as they drank one more glass: "To Mabel."

We even had a genuine Christmas pudding, which was set ablaze in the kitchen. More brandy kept the blue flame flickering and seemed to loosen up already soused tongues. Like me, the guests were stuffed with food. Yet I, too, indulged in a generous helping of "Christmas pud" covered with custard and brandied butter. I undid the buttons of my waistcoat and trousers to accommodate a memorable meal.

The meal officially over, Victoria and I took refuge under a palm tree. We stripped off our woolen Christmas fineries, taking in the leeward breeze to cool our brows, and listened to the Queen's annual Christmas Message on Delmar's short-wave radio. Following a rousing "God Save The Queen" played by the honor guard and accompanied by the strains of a single bagpipe from inside the bungalow, the Queen's speech came across the ether, from half a world away.

Her voice boomed from the house, mixing with our poor reception and the gentle lapping of the waves rushing the beach. She spoke of the increasingly prominent and important role played by women in society—a message that resonated with both of us. I was proud that Victoria was becoming a physician. I wondered how the bastion of ex-army men living in a paradise *sans femme* were taking the directive delivered by their sovereign.

I was looking into Victoria's eyes and suddenly saw them vibrate. At the same time, we felt the earth move. Such were not our emotions, nor the few sips of alcohol. "It's an earthquake," Victoria murmured. It was over in a few seconds. There wasn't a tsunami. We headed to the comfort of our room and the chance for yet another siesta to sleep off a wonderful traditional dinner.

With Christmas behind us, the relaxing days on the beach were dwindling as the exigencies of our resumed medical lives and upcoming exams infiltrated my grey matter. The obligations that awaited us on our return to London wormed into our peaceful slumber. Added to these worries was the news that a Christmas blizzard was dumping over twelve inches of snow and sleet and temperatures of six degrees Fahrenheit were gripping the entire mid-Atlantic coast from Washington, D.C. to beyond New York—and further north.

The storm paralyzed air traffic and closed businesses. The polar freeze gusted between twenty-five and thirty miles per hour as the Arctic front dipped low over the American landmass. Snowdrifts of two to three feet accumulated throughout New York. La Guardia and John F. Kennedy Airports were closed, as were the other major international airports up and down the eastern seaboard. We heard reports on Delmar's radio and saw pictures of paralyzed cities and towns with weather maps showing snow depths in the local paper. Each day brought an additional steady light snow adding to the accumulations.

In Antigua, we visited the BOAC office after Boxing Day, December 26, to find out the status of our flight back to New

York and our connecting flight to London. The young Antiguan woman had no information to give us other than, "All flights are cancelled for now."

We persisted. "But when can we fly back to London? Will air travel have resumed by December 31, in five days? We are doctors and must get back to our work." She could not give us a satisfactory answer, other than, "Perhaps you could fly into Philadelphia or another airport further south if they've cleared the snow by then."

I did not fully understand the effects of a blizzard of this magnitude. I had no idea what resumption of normal life on air travel meant. I understood how a sandstorm grounded flights in Egypt, but these were over in a matter of hours. My badgering drew from her lips the words that I hated most. "Come back tomorrow."

Four days before we were to leave, on Saturday, December 28, and almost packed in anticipation of our departure, Delmar drove us into St. John's. We invaded the deserted BOAC office with our tickets in hand, as if our concerted presence could somehow change providence and clear us for take-off.

"The east-coast airports are partially operating," she said in an encouraging tone, "only BWIA has not been cleared to fly into New York." She hesitated as she observed our despondent rejection. Delmar started to talk with her, reverting to his Caribbean accent from the Queen's English, which seemed to open her receptiveness and widen the options.

"There is a chance that there may be two seats I could use for them on Monday's BOAC flight from Barbados to London, which stops here and in Bermuda," she said as if thinking aloud.

"So why not do that? It'll get the young doctors back to work, without loss of days," he said craftily, leaning on the counter as we stood by. She understood the implications of loss of work.

"Come back in a couple hours," she suggested, "I should have their tickets by then."

With smiles all around and heaps of thank yous, we departed feeling optimistic, victorious. There were advantages to having Delmar negotiate with a fellow Antiguan, and of course to being "young doctors."

We received two tickets: St John's Antigua to London Heathrow, skirting the entire east coast morass.

Victoria and I departed a day early. We sat in the mid-cabin section next to one another, holding hands; Victoria's ring twinkled in the dimmed cabin light. We were anxious to start life together in London—my love and I.

PART II

LONDON

SPRING TO AUTUMN 1968

Why did I love her? Because it was her; because it was me.

—Michel de Montaigne

7

DR. AND MRS. MEGUID

1968–1970

One love is unlike another.
—Diane Enns

With our honeymoon over and back in London, I carried Victoria across the entranceway of our tiny flat. She hooked her arm about my neck, laughingly protesting that she was too heavy, while she kicked off her shoes and I dropped her at my destination—our new double bed. We fell into each other's willing arms.

So began our new life together at 15 Albany Street. It was a cozy little nest—our nest. Small and intimate and meeting my expectations for cheerfulness—sunlight. Without the brightness of daylight, I had withered in Manchester, but in London, the mix of sunshine beaming through the windows and Victoria's magnetic and sensual presence engulfed us in a bubble of euphoria. I felt complete, deeply immersed and secure in a blissful union.

Our London terrace house had a black front door with a traditional brass knocker. We faced the famous White House

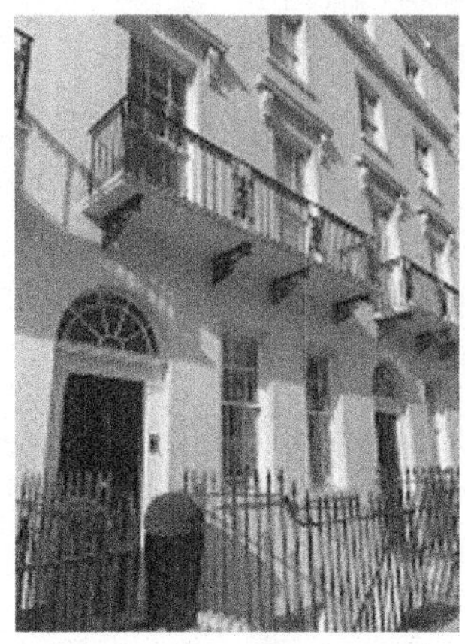

flats across the street and backed onto the splendor of Regent's Park's rose garden. Our furnished flat was an oversized shoebox one flight up. Its front door led down a narrow corridor to a kitchenette past a bathroom with a full-sized tub and a mirror over the sink. Off the corridor was a carpeted living area with a marble-mantled fireplace and lofty floor-to-ceiling window. To the right was our bedroom, with a dresser in front of another floor-to-ceiling window, leaving barely enough room for a double bed and nightstand.

The next few months would be an academically intense time. I had five months of earnest studying, mostly at home, to prepare for the third MB—the General Medical Council's qualifying exams. Success meant I'd be a doctor. Only then would I have time to arrange our London wedding reception, probably in late May. Thereafter, I'd become fully engulfed by my two six-month stints as medical then surgical house officer.

Victoria had to complete her third year of medical school and be promoted to her fourth and last year of school, which was followed by the GMC exam and two-house officer jobs. By the summer of 1970, we could potentially consider training in America.

We became two separate individuals as we drifted from the lushness of love into the dry, impassionate deserts of learning. Our worlds revolved around the life that would ultimately make us physicians. We followed different schedules and worked in different hospitals. The routine of studying engulfed us, sapping our spontaneity and liveliness, leaving us with much less time to focus on each other than we had on our honeymoon. It was going to be a busy and hectic eighteen months.

As a break, we visited Shirley over long weekends, seeking relaxation and intimacy on our beloved Isle. We *could* now share a bed, two study-fatigued bodies lying side by side. We relaxed in the sun in Shirley's garden and sometimes Victoria cooked.

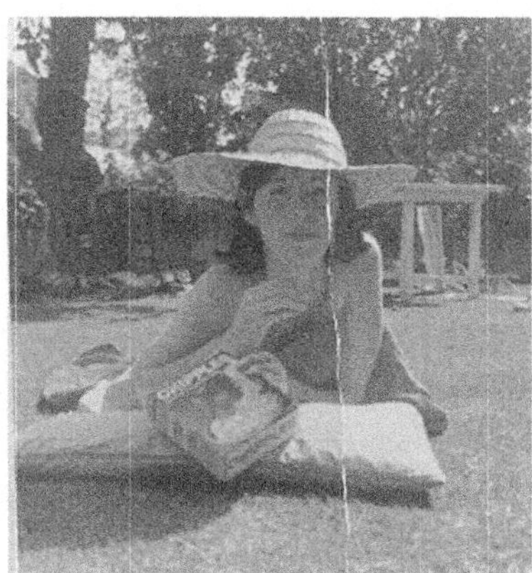

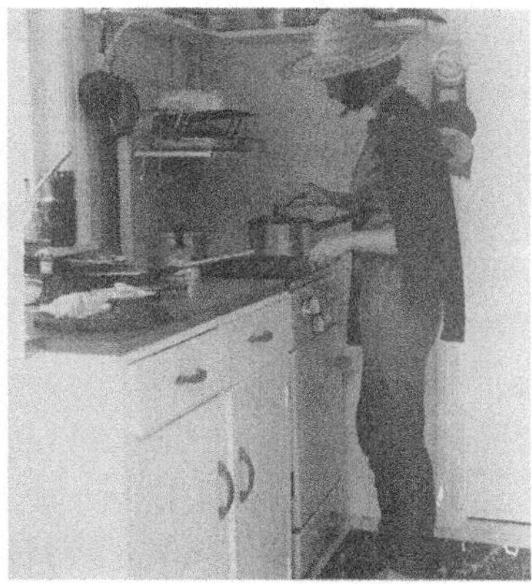

"Shirley, have you seen our marriage certificate?" I asked soon after our return from crossing the Atlantic, holding it out for her to view.

She grasped it in both hands looking it over. "It's probably a fake." Chuckling, she added, "Much nicer to live in sin, after all." She dropped the green-colored document into my hands. What witty or sarcastic retort had I expected?

Even though we were legally married, Shirley did not yet accept me. Like most mothers, she probably did not think me good enough for her daughter and had hoped Victoria would have found a rich, titled Englishman. She could cherish her secret hopes that Victoria, her baby, her precious daughter, could have married anyone in the world, as Shirley would tell me on several occasions. I admired my wife for her fortitude, but at such times I wished she would speak up and defend me.

Despite the implication that our marriage was bogus, Shirley fantasized a grand wedding.

"Darling," she said, addressing Victoria, "I can now arrange for the wonderful reception that you deserve. We'll get you a white dress with a train that extends three to four feet behind you. A ring bearer. Yes, we'll need a cute ring bearer, bridesmaids, and grooms, lots of flowers—and of course a tiara." I could hear the organ music in my head as she spoke, although I could not imagine this glamorous affair going forward. "*All my friends* will be there. We'll have Champagne—lots of it, and canapés heaped with caviar." It sounded grand. And, I liked the idea but how practical was it? Who was going to arrange all this and who was going to pay remained unanswered questions. She looked at her daughter and then at me, sensing our mounting anxiety. "Don't worry about it, darling, I'll arrange everything," she assured her daughter.

Shirley was oblivious to the strains of our eighteen months of demanding academic schedules. Her behavior was familiar to us; Victoria would end up having to salvage the situation. I could see the concern on my wife's face, although she made no effort to contradict or enlighten her mother. Secretly, I thought that Shirley could pull it off, but Victoria showed her apprehension, wondering if her mother would be overwhelmed making the arrangements.

I set up my study schedule for the exam the minute Victoria left for her medical school in the morning. I reasoned that there would be a finite number of practical questions to ask. My gut sense was that the examiners could only compose questions from a predetermined pool of knowledge in each field, from grounds we had covered. These would constitute the essay questions. Working on the assumption that "common things occur commonly," I drew a Gaussian bell curve for the frequency each question had been asked during the past four years, information I culled from past exam papers that were bound in a volume found in the library. A distinct pattern of the most frequently asked questions emerged for each discipline—these were the topics I reviewed first.

I made lengthy lists of all the other topics I would have to study, developing a strategy for answering the essay questions in thirty to forty-five minutes by first writing an outline—a series of headings—and then fleshing them out in essay form. If I ran out of time, the examiner would at least have an idea of what my comprehensive answer would have been. When I finished prioritizing this information, I panicked. It seemed that there were so many topics and not much time.

I had forgotten what a painfully slow reader I was because English was my third language and I had a problem with dyslexia. It was a solitary and boring task to reread my notes to refresh the minutiae. There was some material I did not remember ever having learned in the first place. Within a week, dog-eared books, folders of notes, endless to-do lists tacked onto the curtains and memory lists taped to the mantel piece and bathroom mirror converted our small living room into a jungle of papers taped to the side of our only bookshelf. The mess of notes eventually migrated to the back of the toilet door.

Studying at home was akin to solitary confinement. The days dragged on while Victoria was at the hospital. We lived at a time when conveniences such as cell phones, text messages and emojis didn't exist. I walked through the rose garden in Regent's Park as often as I could to clear my mind and get some cool air. Although my brain felt like a jumbled mush of porridge, seeing and smelling the roses helped consolidate the material I had just read. Occasionally, Victoria gave me a shopping list, and I walked to the Sainsbury market down the road.

On weekends when she was on call in the hospital and when I was anxious about being left alone, I would pack my books and take the bus or train south of London to Blackheath, staying in Mother's empty flat—she was in Egypt, once more. I would walk in Greenwich Park to the Observatory and Maritime Museum. Standing on the heights, I took in the view of London to the north of the Thames. As I walked along the footpaths that meandered among the old oak trees, I thought about the stress of our work and the fatigue it caused. Victoria and I were familiar strangers once more with emotional detachment between us. I could not remember when we were last intimate, had gone out for a meal, or enjoyed some form of entertainment during a weekday. As busy physicians, was this how our married life was going to be?

The remedy was a trip to the Isle of Wight. Shirley made us Friday night dinners and let us sleep late on Saturday mornings. Walking hand in hand along the seawall, we inhaled the ozone-rich wind roaring off the Solent. I felt close to Victoria once more. We used Shirley's car to drive up to the Brading Downs, where we sat and reminded ourselves that despite our busy and divergent schedules, we could still enjoy watching the sunset and remember the tenderness of our love.

8

FINAL MB & APOTHECARIES EXAM

MAY 1968

Spanish rain, A maiden's dress, Apothecary pills, And ancient thrills; Melancholy kills A girl's caress.

—Roman Payne

Once I finished medical school, my £700 scholarship would cease and I would need to make a living. I immersed my being in that singular goal.

The Apothecaries Act of 1815 granted the Royal Apothecary Society the power to certify and regulate medical practitioners throughout England and Wales. I viewed passing this test as my Plan B. Passing the Society of Apothecaries exam would be the insurance necessary to allow me to practice medicine in the UK should I fail the third MB, after almost five years of study. The latter was the *real* thing. With the Apothecary diploma's acronym (LMSSA) behind my name, I could work as a GP while retaking the final MB.

The Apothecaries exam was held in their august banquet hall in Blackfriars. A single proctor placed the exam papers face down on small, flimsy desks set out in rows. There were fewer candidates than I had expected, about two dozen, and none from my class. When the proctor stated that we could start, I turned over the paper and recognized the topics I had studied and the answers that I had prepared. After three hours of writing, I felt I had gone through the wringer. Exhausted, I strolled home—a lengthy walk, even for London. I felt I had done my best.

At 7 a.m. a couple of weeks later, the postman dropped an envelope through the mail slot. I took it up to our flat and placed it next to me as Victoria and I started our breakfast.

"Well, aren't you going to open it?" she asked.

"I'm not sure I want to know the results. Is the Licentiate of the Society so important? What if I didn't pass? Failing the exam will demoralize me and might affect my performance on the final MB."

"After all the studying you did? My darling, *you have such fragile self-esteem.* I have confidence in you. If you've passed," she persisted, "won't it have the opposite effect? I mean, why bother sitting for it if you don't want to know the outcome?"

I picked up my letter opener and sliced the envelope open. Peeking in, I quietly said, "I passed."

"You see. Well done. I've got to go now or I'll be late for my first lecture." With that, she disappeared for the day. I cleared the table and picked up the shopping list.

We should have gone out and celebrated, but the news was anti-climactic. I was not sure if I was going to add the acronym LMSSA behind my name. While I loved the traditional antiquity of the association, strangely, I did not feel more qualified than before passing. Instead, I considered the final MB as the real hurdle. Passing it would announce to the world that I was a genuine, bona fide physician.

In the midst of our "medical business," I had applied for a British passport. A civil servant of Her Majesty's Home Office knocked on the door of 15 Albany Street one Saturday morning. He asked numerous questions about the length of time I had known Victoria, why we had married in Boston, and if indeed we were living together. I signed forms, and satisfied that this was a marriage based on love, the young man departed.

Some days later, my passport arrived. With Victoria sitting on my knee, for we had only one Mission-Style armchair, I admired in awe the much-coveted document that declared me a British subject. We could now travel to almost every country in the world without needing a visa. If only we had the time and money!

Placing her arm around my neck, Victoria beamed with pride. By marriage, she had bestowed on me a liberating gift, one that freed me from the travel limitations imposed by my Egyptian travel document.

The passport was, indeed, one more step in my becoming British. My new passport conferred the security of a British citizen. At the same time, emotionally, I would always consider myself an *Ibn el Balad*—an Egyptian native son. How could I not be? Was there no truth in the saying, "Once you drink from the waters of the Nile, Egypt is always in your blood?"

A few weeks later, I sat for the General Medical Council exams. After three strenuous hours, I exited the exam hall with my brain sapped dry. This set of exams seemed much harder. Had I mentioned *this* or *that* in answer to a question? Following the exam, nightmares woke me.

Before I knew the outcome, we escaped the intensity of our London life by seeking the restorative tranquility of the Isle of Wight. While there, we finalized pared-down reception plans that were far from Shirley's fantasy. Reality was dictated by her checkbook.

With the location of our celebration decided—The Great

Hall of the Worshipful Society of Apothecaries, a benefit of my membership—the question was whether to assume I had passed the GMC's final MB, entitling me to add MBBS to my name and emboss the invitation with the prefix "Doctor," or use my name without such a prefix. Shirley claimed that her daughter had married a "doctor." However, at my insistence, we settled on "Mister," fearing that I would jinx the outcome of the final MB. Imagine writing doctor only to discover that I had failed!

The wedding invitation disturbed me even further since I denied my Egyptian heritage by omitting my father's name on the invitation when I was indeed the late Abdel Aziz's son.

Mrs Robert Perfect
requests the pleasure of your company
on Saturday, 11th May
at 3 o'clock
at Apothecaries' Hall
Blackfriars Lane, Queen Victoria Street, E.C.4
after the marriage of her daughter
Victoria
to
Mr. Marwan Meguid.

R.S.V.P.
Brook,
Seaview,
Isle of Wight

In the midst of worrying about social concerns, a letter arrived from the Egyptian Education Office in Mayfair. The director had received permission from the Mogamma to add the United States into my Egyptian passport. What? Seven months later? I telephoned the secretary. "Thank you so much, but my plans have changed. I am no longer interested in going to America; after all, I applied some time ago."

He seemed perplexed, "Do come. It might be useful at a future date."

I thanked him for his trouble and said again, "I've got too much work here." As I hung up, I thought about the difference between Western and Egyptian bureaucracy and culture. With my trip to Boston and potential American job offers, the issue of my identity would become even more complicated. Where did my loyalties lie? My identity was confused.

In the midst of our planning, a letter arrived notifying me that I had successfully passed the GMC's final MB examination, crowning my often anxious and challenging passage through medical school. I had received a first-class education at a respected London institute and could now call myself Dr. Meguid with a great sense of accomplishment. I had achieved the "label" my headmaster in Manchester had alluded to some years previously. There was no congratulatory card or even a letter of maternal wisdom from Mother. I did, however, receive my first UK malpractice insurance invoice for £2.

Our wedding reception was a classic English affair held on a gloriously sunny May afternoon. Our guests streamed into the grand Apothecaries' Hall, which was festooned with the gilded frames of ancient dignitaries hung on polished oak-paneled walls between magnificent stained-glass windows. Victoria's relatives, many of our medical school friends, my German family—Oma, Mother, Gulnar and Freimut and their two youngsters—and Onkel Hansi and Tante Trudel and their daughter, friends of Mother's, attended.

None of my Egyptian family came; my Egyptian grandparents had passed, and my maiden aunts couldn't travel without the permission of one of my uncles. It would be difficult for them to find the money and almost impossible to obtain a visa within a reasonable time.

The new Mrs. Meguid looked sensual and sublime, a delicate, timeless English beauty in a sleeveless green silk dress with a high neckline and falling just below her knees—my goddess. I wore my dark pinstriped suit with a silver silk tie and a boutonnière pinned on by Victoria.

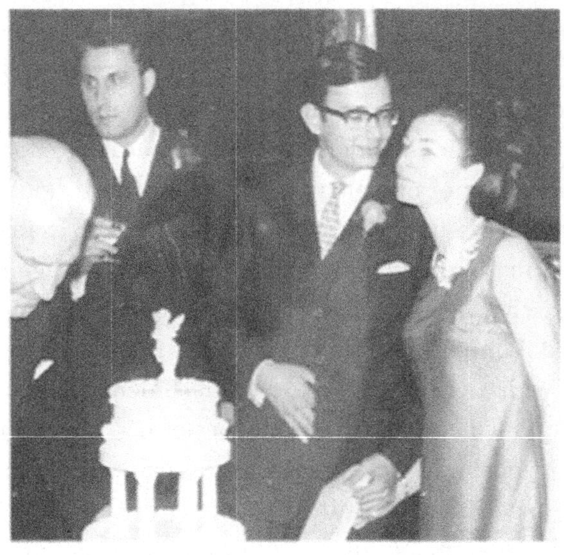

Champagne flowed freely, and white-gloved butlers in black tie passed exquisite canapés on silver platters. Per custom, Shirley had baked the top of a three-tiered wedding cake in the traditional British fruitcake, consisting of the juice and zest of oranges and lemons, ground almonds, chopped hazelnuts, walnuts, pecans, and more than a pound of assorted dried apricots, figs, prunes, and candied glacé cherries, all soaked with the finest whiskey and covered in a layer of marzipan—just what I loved. The guests ate the frosted sponge cake that formed the other two tiers.

Freimut, ever his gregarious self, was the master of ceremony. He stood on a chair, humorously addressing us. I had prepared some remarks: notes of gratitude to our mothers, followed by my waving our American marriage certificate to assure the gathering that Victoria and I were indeed wed, albeit in Boston. Uncle John made some suitable remarks concerning his brilliant and beautiful niece.

Shirley was down—sitting in a window seat waiting for the younger generation to engage her in chat or banter. She seemed overwhelmed at the loss of her daughter. Mother was up—chatting merrily with the company of German family and friends who attended the reception. The German relatives stood around, unfamiliar with the etiquette and formality of English receptions and hindered by a language barrier. The Brits, including Victoria's friends and relatives, drank freely and chatted among themselves, ignoring the Germans who they had been at war with twenty years earlier. Most of our medical school friends, among them John Rackey, Jonathan Marrow and Kanti Rajani, were unfamiliar with the customs of either group and, hence, chatted about the recent exams.

Perhaps dancing would have bridged the cultural gap. The mainstay of Egyptian weddings was a musical ensemble and belly dancing. It remains unclear to me whether the lack of music was because of Shirley's economic considerations or my oversight. In the upheaval of making the reception arrangements, I forgot to arrange for a formal photographer—a sad omission.

Following the reception, most of the guests made their way to Mother's flat in Blackheath, where a German-style evening buffet was served.

According to tradition, the wedding cake top was preserved once it was considered sufficiently imbued with the praiseworthiness of its expensive whiskey, to be served and savored by discerning, deserving family members with a decent cup of tea one year later.

9

THE INTERVIEW

MAY 1968

Early experiences of lack of belonging and acceptance can promote unhealthy shame experiences that can manifest as a sense of being essentially unworthy, unlovable, and bad.

—Kathy L. Kain and Stephen J. Terrell

As a full-fledged physician, I was proud of my achievements. I had been shaped into a knowledgeable individual and, like my classmates, had survived the demanding schedule. We had absorbed the subtle changes of clothing and attitude necessary for a medical transformation.

The final phase of my formal medical education lay ahead. I had to put into practice what I had learned by fulfilling the General Medical Council's requirement for a six-month medical and six-month surgical house officer's job—a supervised internship. I felt that the odds of successfully applying for my first clinical job at UCH stood a chance.

However, global politics and old conflicts had flared and come once again to England—and the university—with great anger and anti-immigrant sentiments. In response to the June 1967 Arab–Israeli Six-Day War, passions between the student's Zionist community and the Arab students in London flared up. There were pitched battles in the University Union that deteriorated into furniture throwing. These public demonstrations of anger solved no problem; they only reinforced entrenched opinions.

The other international event that year was the influx into Britain of young Commonwealth immigrants, including many well-qualified professionals and their families from East Africa. At the turn of the century, the British colonial powers ruling East Africa had encouraged the migration of Indian bureaucrats to form a distinct middle class—a buffer between the indigenous population and the British ruling elite. Their ancestors considered England home, and to prove it, they had British passports stating they were Her Majesty's subjects, just like me.

Following their independence from Britain, the national governments of Uganda, Malawi and other African nations evicted the Indians during the mid- to late sixties. About 50,000 immigrants arrived annually in the United Kingdom. It was not uncommon to encounter Indian bus conductors who had PhDs but who had not yet found an appropriate job or had yet to assimilate into the British workforce. Similarly, East African Indian physicians immigrated to Britain and got junior registrar or junior resident positions. They accepted such professional demotions to gain entrance into the National Health Service.

Enoch Powell, the xenophobic Conservative Member of Parliament for Wolverhampton, said that if this inflow was the "material of the future growth of the immigrant-descended population," the character and culture of Britain would change irrevocably. The groundswell of anti-immigrant sentiment was exacerbated by Mr. Powell's inflammatory political speech in 1968, projecting that "the black man will have the whip hand over the white man." Quoting from Virgil's *Aeneid,* he concluded, "I seem to see 'The River Tiber foaming with much blood.'" Powell's speech was highly publicized, tapped into the English working population's collective fear, and bolstered British public prejudice. Did the phobia extend to educated physicians? Based on the reaction I received after my election to the chairman position of the Physiology Society, it well could have been. Of greater concern for me was that these experienced physicians competed directly with the annual tide of newly qualified British-trained physicians.

An appointment as a house surgeon or physician in one's teaching hospital was a propitious career step on the academic ladder. I had expected to apply to a house surgeon's job on the surgical unit with Professor Pilcher, but his retirement and the failure to appoint a timely successor derailed this aspect of my career plan. With the surgical unit in flux and engulfed by leadership uncertainty, I decided to pursue a house physician appointment first.

Professor Rosenheim's star had risen to national eminence. During the years I had progressed in medical school, our paths occasionally crossed. He would acknowledge me with a nod and a smile of recognition. I continued to attend his medical rounds from time to time, and I concluded that he remembered me.

I felt a kinship with Professor Rosenheim, for despite the differences in our background, surely, he had struggled. Professor Rosenheim's parents, Jews, had fled their hometown because of the fear of persecution and had sought refuge in England. Like me, the young Max Rosenheim must have had to face the same prejudice and problems as a foreigner during his school days, he as a Jew, I as an Arab. He had also gone to Massachusetts General Hospital in Boston for further studies. I admired him as the paragon of medical and professional respectability—the academic I wanted to emulate.

In May of 1968, I saw in the *British Medical Journal* that Professor Rosenheim was advertising an opening for his six-month house physician job. I applied, believing that the sum of my additional clinical locums, my diligent application for numerous prize exams, winning the Erichsen Award in Surgery and my elective in Boston would prove enticing credentials to warrant his consideration as a suitable candidate, a fledgling physician he could mentor and mold. Young and enthusiastic, I had not yet come across the cynical attitude among medical students that one only gets a job on a professorial service by PR (per rectum) or PV (per vaginum): kissing his ass or fucking his daughter.

Within forty-eight hours of my application, I received an invitation for an interview. I was surprised but delighted. He could have refused to interview me. Maybe Professor Rosenheim would appreciate my credentials, and no doubt, he had made a few telephone calls to my in-house referees, primarily Dr. Gerald Stern.

I arrived a few minutes early and waited outside his office door in a quietly buoyant mood. After a short wait, I was motioned into the office. Professor Rosenheim sat behind a high table, looking down on me with my student file open in front of him. Two assistants sat on either side; all four had various shades of dark complexions—physicians recently displaced from Idi Amin's Uganda. I looked up at them, encouraged that Professor Rosenheim, the exemplar of meritocracy and now President of the Royal College of Physicians, must be a decent, tolerant man for taking in physicians who had fled persecution in Africa.

Professor Rosenheim wore a dark blue suit and a waistcoat with a gold watch chain strung across his chest. Below the table, at my eye level, I saw his chubby legs crossed at his ankles, exposing highly polished Oxford lace-ups and dark socks that ended a few inches below the trouser turn-ups, revealing pale, hairless legs.

He barely looked up from the papers as he started his interrogation.

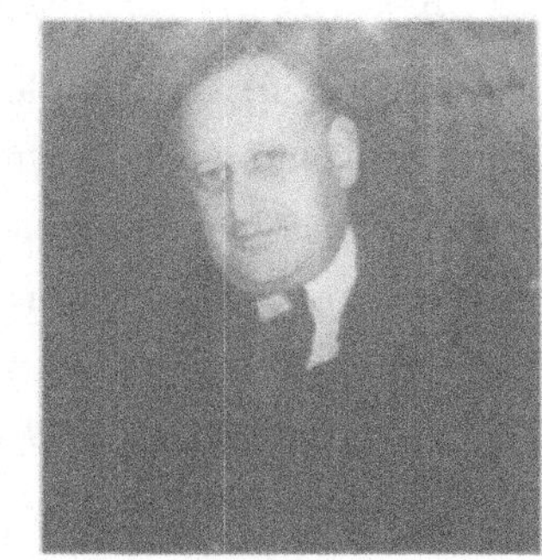

"What is your name?"

"Marwan Abdel Meguid."

"Where do you come from?" His tone was cold—so different from the warmth he affected on rounds. His question threw me off balance. My records were right in front of him.

"Egypt," I replied apprehensively.

Without hesitation, he said, "Go back there. You're not welcome here."

He closed my file and rose.

I was stunned into speechlessness. I sat motionless trying to take in—to process—what I had just heard. *You're not welcome here.*

Why had he invited me for an interview? I fumed with rage. I wanted to yell *you* of all people, *you* who have found a safe haven and fame in England, *you* the recipient of heaped accolades, *you* are discriminating against *me, a little student*? Despite his many worldly honors and greatness, his behavior as a mere fellow human was unbelievable and abhorrent.

I seethed with fury at my dismissal. I felt betrayed by him, by the medical profession and by the very institute that had trained me—I was dismissed, cast out worse than a dirty dog—scorned as a human being.

Walking the short distance home along Euston Road toward our flat, I howled aloud with pain to the dismay of passersby. I wanted retribution for being invited merely to be slaughtered—yet I had no recourse.

Ancient wounds simmering just below the surface

reopened and seized me again. I was transported back to that helpless little boy abandoned by my mother, not wanted and then as now without remedy; branded a failure at eleven by my father and feeling wretched for being so undesirable —*unworthy and bad.* I wanted to crawl under Oma's vast skirt, seeking protection and security from a hostile world—from the woman who loved me and who was my true mother.

I yearned for comfort and consolation from my wife. I wanted and needed her reassurance—to hold me, to tell me that it's alright, that I'm a good man, and that she loved and cared for me, that she understood the *root cause* of my pain—to sooth and comfort me. I expected no less.

I got home, smarting from the humiliation and shame. I had a gargantuan wound, a slash with a scimitar from head-to-toe, gushing blood. I needed Victoria—to soothe my pain, kiss my wound, restore my confidence in humanity and heal me.

She looked up from her books. "Well? How did it go? No doubt you got the job."

I blurted out the events, banging my fist on the table. "No, no. That motherfucker told me to go back to Egypt and that I'm not welcome in England."

Victoria continued sitting and looking up at me, and after a moment's hesitation, shrugged her shoulders and said, "Never mind. It's just a job interview. There'll be plenty more."

Standing in front of her in a state of incomprehension, I was unable to say a word. I stared at her from my place in the emotional wilderness: not accepted, not belonging, and wondering where Victoria stood.

Was she blind to Rosenheim's profound prejudice? Was she unaware of the gaping wound he had inflicted? How could Victoria not understand my despair? Was she too preoccupied with her studies to recognize my pain, or was she afraid to indulge my emotional baggage? Did she understand present-day English culture so much better than I did?

All I know, looking back to that fateful day some fifty years ago, is that her inability to acknowledge my pain seemed to marked a turning point between us—she had broken our bond. At that instant, I saw her as the aloof white English woman and I was, yet again that fucking foreigner, standing on the opposite side of the divide. I was her stranger. She became mine. I would find no empathy here.

10

THE WOUNDED PHOENIX

JULY 1968

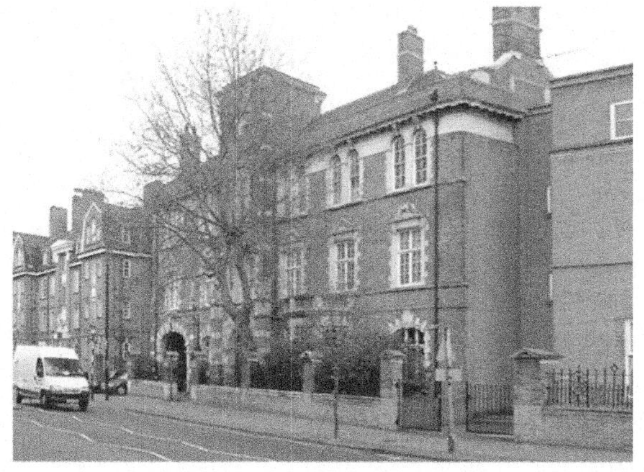

In the depths of winter,
I finally learned that within me there lay an invincible summer.
—Albert Camus

Because of the repudiation from Rosenheim, I worked tirelessly to find a job. I checked the notice board at UCH, flicked through the jobs section of journals, and inquired among my peers. After a week, I saw an advertisement for house physicians at Bethnal Green Hospital, a district hospital in the heart of the tough cockney neighborhood of London's East End. It stated that "successful applicants would be suitably matched to one of three available jobs." Since Bethnal Green was in St. Bartholomew's sphere of influence, Roger, my St. Bartholomew's friend with whom I reviewed anatomy while we lived together at Commonwealth Hall, told me that it was unlikely they would take a UCH graduate.

I needed a job to restore my confidence as an able physician. In the absence of UCH-affiliated job openings at the Whittington Hospital in North London, Bethnal Green was my next best bet, if for no other reason than to practice my interview skills.

The Tube took me from Great Portland Street station to Bethnal Green, where I surfaced onto Cambridge Heath Road. A short walk later, I gazed at the wrought iron gates of the hospital's administrative building. Young Bart's graduates packed the waiting room. The only remaining chair was in the corner by the door. I was ignored by everyone except the crewmembers of their medical school's eight, who nodded cordially. The atmosphere was jovial. They bantered, dropping names of physicians at Bethnal Green that they knew, mentioning their daddies, and deciding among themselves who would get which job. Roger was right; I had the wrong school tie. I decided to go home to avoid another humiliation.

As I rose to sneak out, the boardroom door opened, and my name was called. Twelve eyes weighed me up as I entered. I sat opposite Dr. Silber, a portly gerontologist of a ten-bed unit, who wore an unconventional mustard tweed suit complementing his shock of silver hair. His partner, Dr. Gilliland, an internist with piercing green eyes and a welcoming smile, was attired in sober gray.

"Have you cared for elderly patients?" Dr. Silber asked. The stale smell of urine with endless cries of "nurse" from bedridden patients jumped to mind.

I had managed acutely ill hospitalized elderly patients despite my aversion to decrepit end-of-lifers. So technically I considered the answer to be truthfully in the affirmative. "Yes," I said dryly, although not altogether convincingly.

He was unswayed, but persisted in trying to generate a spark of enthusiasm. "My patients are in their sixties and seventies, mainly women with chronic illnesses, mostly heart conditions admitted for a tune-up." He stared at me and hesitated. "They have their meds adjusted, just like re-winding a toy before being discharged. You'll arrange meals on wheels and so on, but Sister and her nurses are super at doing all that. We'll follow them in the clinic. Some may need re-admitting six to eight weeks later. You'll do daily rounds with Sister, and we'll do rounds weekly. It's rather fun."

I nodded. *Fun! Really?* Now I imagined a dreaded nursing home—the repository of abandoned elders. Where was the acute medical care? I needed to put my book knowledge into action. Dr. Gilliland spoke up, "I see you've spent some time at Mass General Hospital in Boston. You won a travel scholarship from the British Medical Association. Did you enjoy America?" In my peripheral vision, several heads along the long interview table nodded in approval.

"It was a very intense six weeks," I said. "I learned a great deal and enjoyed caring for my acutely sick patients."

His eyes smiled. "Isn't it an exciting town? I, too, was at Mass General many years ago." He had the prestigious BTA. I felt an immediate affinity to him; I had probably walked in his footsteps on the wards.

Dr. Gilliland was a quiet, unassuming man gifted with great personal charm. He had been a medic with the commandos during the war in then-Palestine and retained his military bearing. He was born in Rhodesia of mixed North Irish and Scottish stock, the son of a member of the pioneer column sent by Rhodes to colonize Moshanaland in 1890 and had received his medical education in Edinburgh.

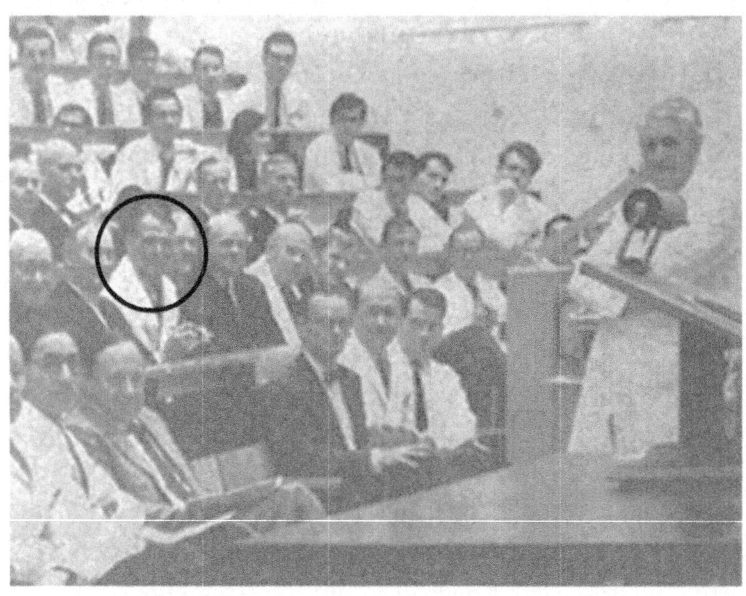

Professor Rosenheim, unknown and Dr. Ian Gilliland. Courtesy of the British Medical Journal

His features were soft and welcoming. "I'm also a consultant at the Hammersmith Postgraduate Hospital"—a prestigious institute—"and, as you can imagine, I'm interested in teaching the junior staff. We'd be doing rounds twice a week and seeing patients in clinic together once a week." These words were music to my ears, for UCH had given me a solid medical foundation but I needed mentoring, especially by an accomplished general physician.

"I have a medical unit of twenty-four acutely sick patients, including heart disease, thyroid problems and diabetes. I also have one or two morbidly obese women on a total starvation diet. They are innovative medical challenges. Isn't that interesting?"

"How fascinating," I replied. "These metabolic-nutritional problems appeal to me." He had the jewels that I sought—twenty-four acute care medical beds. Before I could say another word, he looked at Dr. Silber and offered me the job.

I rode the Tube back to Regent's Park. I felt alive, imbued with a sense of validation. I wanted to stand up in the middle of the swaying carriage and shout to my fellow riders, I'm not a reject. I matter. I'm not *unworthy.* I have a job!" At the same time, I felt some ambivalence; had I accepted any job—perhaps a second-rate job at a second-rate hospital—just to feel needed? At first, I was not sure, but I sensed that Dr. Gilliland was a genuine, compassionate man and that he would be a great teacher based on his interests in endocrinology and metabolism.

"I got the job," I declared joyfully on entering our living room. Victoria sat at the table in front of the window with her books and notes, the same table I had sat at cramming a year ago for my finals. I stood behind her, "I got the job," I repeated more soberly waiting for some gratifying comment. Looking up she said, "I haven't heard of Bethnal Green Hospital." After musing for a while, she turned to me and said in lighter banter, "You know it's in the East End—cockney land. You'll soon be talking their dialect."

I attributed her lack of enthusiasm or inquisitiveness about the job to her preoccupation with the workload of her final year at Westminster Hospital, remembering my similarly preoccupied time last year. I quietly wished her response could have been warmer, more vocal and demonstrative; after all, my first job was a monumental event and she would face this situation herself next year.

Maybe, on this occasion, we should have celebrated—to crown my dream of becoming a physician. We should have arranged to go out and had a nice dinner with wine, relaxed together taking stock of our relationship. I've always regretted that I did not take the initiative—nor did she. Instead, we did not even have a celebratory kiss. We stayed home; she studied and I packed.

On Saturday, heading out the door to move into the residential quarters at Bethnal Green Hospital, I kissed Victoria goodbye, once more on the offered cheek.

"Good luck," she said, sensing that I was tense. I knew she meant it. She wished me well, pleased to see me start my career.

Riding in the Tube, I thought about our marriage. Our lives together as young *professionals* was progressing in the right direction, although finding time and creating a mood to be together was becoming a challenge. But our relationship was confusing—hardly the roaring success I wanted.

I missed her attention and our intimacy. Maybe my absence at Bethnal Green would give her more space, or even make us yearn for each other as we did in the early days of our relationship or recently when I was in Boston. Surely, she too must miss our closeness?

Bethnal Green represented a new phase in my life. I was proud of my elevation to a position of responsibility—just like six years ago when I was selected to be a Prefect at Burnage Grammar School after my disastrous first year in Manchester.

Now I felt like an adult, even though I was anxious that I succeed in my first job. Failure in my performance was not out of the question, yet it wasn't an option.

11

BED REST

Our own body possesses a wisdom which we who inhabit the body lack.

—Henry Miller

To acquaint myself with my patients and to introduce myself to Dr. Gilliland's and Dr. Silber's staff, I started rounds on Sunday morning when the hospital activity was less than during a working day and the stillness on the ward wouldn't be disturbed until visitors began arriving after 4 p.m. I would be on call for emergency medical admissions on Sunday night. I didn't anticipate any.

Wearing a crisp, newly starched white coat with a stethoscope stuffed in one pocket and an emergency medical manual in the other, I thought I looked entirely professional as I strode onto the medical ward to meet Sister Ryan and her nurses. Sister wore the dark blue uniform commensurate with her senior status, her uniform crowned with her nursing school cap. Her competence and demeanor were typical of the Irish nurses who had graduated from the nursing school at Bethnal Green.

Accompanied by Sister Ryan's staff nurse, we started with the bed closest to the nursing station and walked along one row of twelve beds, then crossed over to the other side of the ward and came back along the other twelve beds to the ward's entrance and Sister's office. Beside each patient, she said in a soft authoritative voice, "This is Dr. Meguid, your new physician. He's taking over your care, so I'll tell him a little bit about you." She sketched a history of each patient's ailment and treatment plan, all the while weighing me up. I was conscious that the staff nurse was eyeing me too.

". . . Mrs. Baker has angina and is undergoing tests. We want her to rest in bed. Miss Shaw, our special Rita, who is fourteen, has newly diagnosed Type 1 diabetes, and we're teaching her to inject insulin to regulate her blood sugar," adding in a whisper as she turned away from the patient, "it's difficult since her family is not very accepting of her condition." I made courteous comments or gestures of acknowledgments while taking notes, grateful for the insights that were delivered in a robust Irish drawl.

We approached a middle-aged man. "Mr. O'Connor is one of our favorites," she said. "He's about to be discharged after resting his heart for the last six weeks following an acute heart attack." As she reached his bed, she said, "This is our new doctor. We've heard many good things about him," and, as if to reassure him, she continued, "but you're going home today when the missus comes. You'll be seeing him for follow-up in the clinic with Dr. Gilliland.

You've done well, and you'll be all right," she intoned, and ended with the Irish proverb, "Remember there's nothing so bad that it can't be worse." He nodded quietly, allowing himself a slight smile.

"You mean, Sister, he's been in the hospital for six weeks and on complete bed rest?"

"Yes. On total bed rest and he's done well," she replied.

"No problems with deep venous thrombosis?"

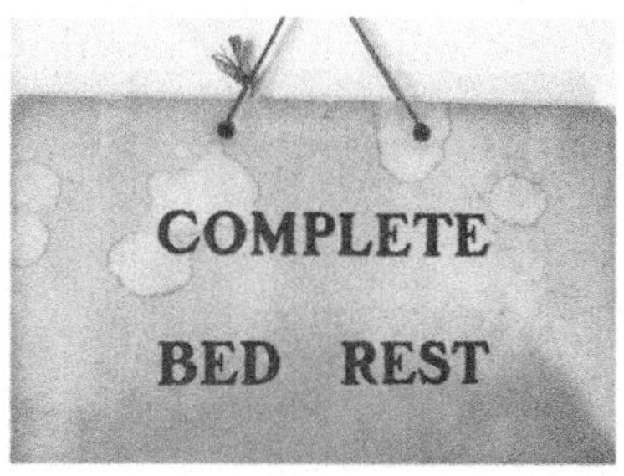

"Oh, no. He just rested and has done well." As she talked, my mind went back some fourteen years to the day in Cairo when my father's body arrived in its simple pine coffin from Beirut.

I was nearly twelve when he was hospitalized at the American University Hospital for pneumonia and pleurisy. As my father lay in bed, he wrote every day chronicling his hospital course. The letters, numbered sequentially, arrived the next morning in Cairo, and Mother would read them to us when we came home from school. In the first, he related "difficulty taking my breath." The second claimed "ease in breathing after fluid on my lungs was drained." In all his letters, he also claimed to suffer from fatigue and exhaustion—a common symptom in heart failure, as I was to learn on the wards at UCH. In his third letter, he complained of a burning sensation in his left calf. Hearing Mother read this aloud, I didn't understand that his new symptom portended disaster. He chose not to report its progression to a dull ache with swelling of his calf to his physician, fearing that this would postpone his planned discharge on the tenth hospital day.

As I had learned at UCH, clots formed in the deep calf veins during bed rest. In some patients, they grew like a knotted rope, going up the vein of the leg, causing symptoms of burning in the calf with an ache and heavy sensation in the leg. When the clot was disturbed by activity, it could break loose from its attachment to the vein wall and travel into the lungs, leading to death from a pulmonary embolus, which shut down oxygen to the brain and the rest of the body. It was a relatively common plague for the bedridden sick as well as pregnant and post-partum mothers. Since my father had not complained of the symptoms, the diagnosis was not made, and heparin therapy was not given. Neither in my father's case nor that of Mr. O'Connor was early ambulation considered, and I wondered about the different outcomes.

Sister's voice brought me back to the present. A fuss occurred behind us: Rita was wobbling out of bed. Steadying her back to the edge of the bed, I noted glassy eyes and beads of sweat. *What should I do?* The staff nurse reappeared with a glass of orange juice, "Here Rita, sip this," as she held the glass to her lips. Within seconds, the patient came around, her eyes focused on us, color returned and sweating stopped.

Sister asked, "Did you give yourself too much insulin this morning, Rita? We'll go over the dosing schedule shortly. Now you rest." We resumed our rounds.

Apart from Mr. O'Connor and another cardiac patient, the rest of my patients were women. Up to this point, I had never managed any of these "bread and butter" conditions on my own, and I began to worry if I was up to the task, particularly because Sister had endorsed me so generously.

Of the twenty-four patients in the ward, three rested on my mind the most. Mrs. Sloan was a slender, older woman with an emotionless affect, suffering from rheumatoid arthritis. She sat in an armchair next to her bed, legs crossed, passively looking me up and down while Sister sketched a thumbnail of her condition. Nothing much had been done for her during her month-long stay, which mystified me since this condition did not seem to warrant hospitalization. Was I missing something?

"What are we doing for her?"

Stepping away from the bed, Sister said, "You'll have to ask Dr. Warren, her consultant."

"Dr. Warren? I thought Dr. Gilliland was the head of this ward."

"Yes. Dr. Warren runs the rheumatology clinic and occasionally admits his patients on your service. You'll have to care for her in consultation with him."

My initial misgivings about this job stirred once more. It seemed I had other consultants to whom I would report.

A few beds along, Mrs. Jenkins, originally from Jamaica, smiled and greeted me warmly. "Yes," she said, confirming Sister's account, "I've lost eighty pounds in the last three months." She had weighed almost three hundred and sixty pounds when Dr. Gilliland admitted her. Turning her back toward the patient, Sister said, embarrassed and smiling, in a lowered voice, "We had to use the scale on the loading dock."

Mrs. Jenkins was on a total starvation diet apart from daily vitamins and drinking water and was allowed up to three hundred calories per day if she had the desire to eat. She was one of the morbidly obese patients Dr. Gilliland had mentioned.

"How are you feeling? Hungry?" I asked.

"No. The longer I don't eat, the less hungry I am. The problem is, doctor, my weight loss has slowed down, and I want to lose more weight to surprise my man when he returns from Jamaica." Her metabolic condition intrigued me—I had plenty of reading ahead of me when I got back to my room.

The other cardiac patient, Mr. Gupta, a transplant from Madras, was twenty-eight years old and had cardiomegaly, a grossly enlarged heart due to cardiac amyloidosis. The starch-like protein, amyloid, is not consumed by the body and collects between the healthy cells of the heart, liver, kidneys, spleen, and other tissues. In his case, it was deposited primarily between his cardiac fibers, grossly enlarging his heart and causing it to pump ineffectively. There was no curable treatment for his condition, which resulted in early death due to congestive heart failure and arrhythmias. Mr. Gupta sat propped up in bed, grasping the railings and fighting for air. He reached anxiously out to me and grabbed my arm as he panted. His hand was sweaty, and his eyes were begging me to help him. Alarmed, my first response was that I had no idea how to help him, and then, common sense kicked in.

"Let's get him a humidifier oxygen mask. Give him some theophylline to open his airways, 5 mg morphine, subcutaneous, to ease his anxiety."

"Anything else?" Sister asked.

"I'll review his cardiac meds after rounds."

The staff nurse fluffed his pillows and helped him sit up more in bed to ease his breathing. The flashback of my difficulty in breathing as a toddler when I was in Cairo and I had whooping cough, that feeling of asphyxiating, of being hungry for air and fearful of dying rushed over me. A powerful memory—one second, no breath, and death.

Sister invited me for a cup of tea and a dry, bland homemade tea biscuit. Several young Irish graduates from the nursing school joined us. Sister gave the introductions; the beguiling nurse with an appealing smile and flirtatious stare was Hanna. The tea trolley lady and the nursing orderlies who I would see daily on the ward were also present. The atmosphere was cordial as we sipped our steaming teas. Sister informally but selectively shared concerns about patients and their families, including issues relating to the staff, all the while as her protégées conversed in murmurs among themselves.

Following tea, I read charts and then chatted with the

patients to gain a more thorough understanding of their complaints, examined each of them to confirm their diagnoses and wrote a summary in their chart. As I saw one patient after another, I became apprehensive about how I would manage twenty-four patients on my own. The staff nurse, Hanna, shadowed me, looking on curiously. When I turned to her, she offered missing patient data or an answer when a difficult issue arose. Out of the corner of my eye, I noted that she slowly crept closer to me with each patient I examined and looked long moments at me until I caught her, after which she would avert her gaze.

I suggested the nurses weigh Mrs. Jenkins every day. I made a huge graph plotting her daily weight loss, which Hanna pinned above her bed while Sister looked on. My intuition was that if we allowed her to have meals on Sunday, the food would rev up her metabolism and ultimately speed weight loss during the following six days when she was fasting.

Mr. Gupta's condition was unsettling and caused me great angst, probably because I knew so little about it. The morphine and oxygen eased Mr. Gupta's apprehension, while the anxiety in his eyes receded. He closed them and rested. I placed his disease on my reading list, while the current management of Mrs. Sloan's rheumatoid arthritis remained an enigma. I planned to consult with Dr. Warren the following morning.

The medical challenges were interesting and my initial apprehension of not knowing how to treat my patients was beginning to recede. Bethnal Green was the right fit for me after all.

12

A DIGNIFIED DEATH

Life is nothing but a continuing dance of birth and death, a dance of change.

Tibetan Book of Living and Dying

On my way to the geriatric unit, a stout, grandmotherly-type woman stepped out of the boardroom and asked if I wanted lunch, because at two, they would stop serving. It was only then that I realized how hungry I was. As I sat alone at the long conference table covered with a white cloth, she served me a delicious Sunday lunch of roast beef, roasted potatoes, Yorkshire pudding and gray-green beans, all swimming in brown gravy. For dessert, I had treacle pudding with plenty of custard and a fresh cup of tea. I ate in silence.

Over the rim of my teacup, I observed slumped bodies in flowered armchairs reading the Sunday paper, while others, paper in hand, had been lulled into sleep. I would get to know these physicians, my colleagues, in the days ahead.

Sister McGrady staffed the geriatric unit, a smaller, more intimate environment on the second floor. She was a very-much-in-charge supervisor, a thin, energetic woman not prone to smiling. She gave me low-key yet definitive guidance concerning each patient—all women—but did not encourage me to examine them because they were having their afternoon rest. By now, I was also beginning to feel the soporific effects of the generous, uncustomary lunch. I decided that Sister McGrady was sufficiently in command of Dr. Silber's patients to allow me to have the pleasure of a postprandial snooze, rationalizing that I was going to be on call that night.

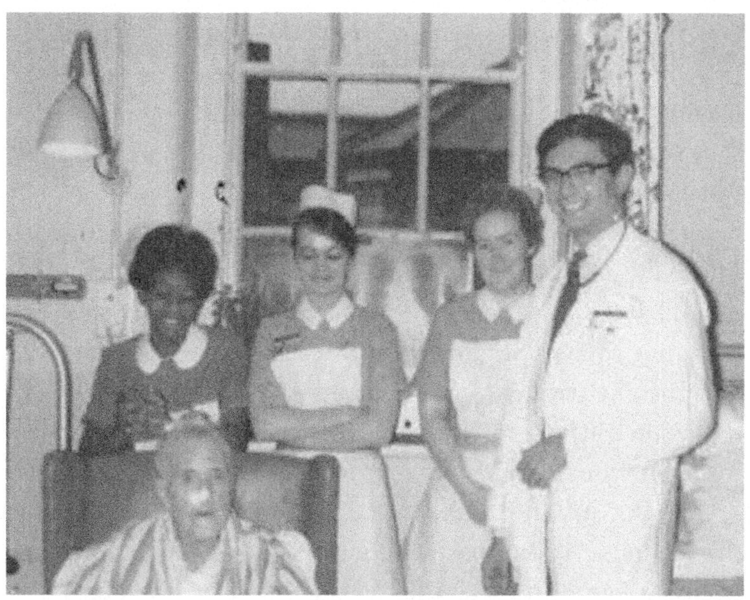

Dr. Meguid with nurses and a geriatric patient

Shortly after I lay down in my new on-call room, Sister McGrady telephoned. "Doctor, you had better come. Mrs. Critchley is dying."

"Dying? Of what? How do you know?"

She repeated, "She's dying. Come on up."

"Please hook her up to an EKG machine. I'm on my way."

When I arrived, it seemed like nothing in the ward had changed. It still was tranquil, and each patient was dozing. The nurses and aides were busy with their duties. Unlike emergency room deaths or those on the surgical ward, there was no hustle and bustle. It looked like death was a daily and undramatic event—as common as a cup of tea.

Mrs. Critchley lay peacefully serene, eyes closed, her face ashen. Salt and pepper hair fanned out on the white pillows that propped her up.

"She's had long-standing heart disease," Sister McGrady said as we gathered around her bed.

"How do you know she's dying?" I whispered, feeling the patient's pulse, terrified that her imminent death was a mistake. Having seen many patients open their eyes and move about as they woke up from anesthesia, I wondered if this patient would wake up.

A nurse drew the curtain about the patient's bed and us. Sister McGrady proceeded to instruct me on the signs surrounding natural death. "First, listen to their lungs for diminishing, shallow, breathing sounds. Second, when listening to the heart, the beats will become irregular." She demonstrated each action, stethoscope stuck in her ear, lightly laying its bell on the patient, hesitating, then shifting it as she listened to these two organs.

Picking up an ophthalmoscope, she proceeded with her instructions. "Look into their pupils. They should react sluggishly to light. Note that the red cells stack up like pennies in the blood vessels at the back of the eyes." As she spoke, I emulated her. It was a comfort to concur with her findings. The sight of the red cells stacking up was remarkable. I'd never seen this before. Sister McGrady was a sharp cookie for her age—

probably late fifties or early sixties. Her disposition suited this job and, no doubt, Dr. Silber's temperament.

"Lastly, look at their hands, which will be cool and pale, while the nails will show signs of blue cyanosis. Be sure to insert their dentures, for once rigor mortis sets in, you'll not be able to pry their jaw apart."

"How long does dying take?" I asked apprehensively.

She looked at me as if to say *did they not teach you youngsters anything in the ivory towers*? Calmly, she announced, "Until the good Lord calls them." Then sighing, she added, "Maybe up to forty-five minutes."

She saw my surprise. "Well, Mrs. Critchley is in her eighties and has lived on her own for some years—no close family, grandchildren, neighbors, or friends, poor ducky. Dr. Silber has cared for her off and on. We expected this event."

"Do I call him?'

"No, I'll do that, and I'll call her son, who works on an oil rig out at sea. You've got to certify her death."

"I see. Let me examine her again to be sure."

Accustomed to relatively rapid "surgical deaths" and to the dramatic ones I had witnessed in casualty, I was uncertain about "medical deaths." The idea that the patient would die during a forty-five-minute period was unsettling. How was Sister McGrady *so* certain?

The only way for me to learn was to draw up a chair and keep running a one-minute EKG strip every few minutes, sensing that an electronic record could not fail me or let me down or even make a mistake. The strip confirmed progressively fewer heartbeats, with irregular or extra beats thrown in from time to time due to irritation of the cardiac muscles. By EKG, death is definite.

Sister was right. After about thirty minutes, the QRS-complexes, representing cardiac contraction, became smaller, indicating a failing, weaker heart with fewer and fewer beats until a flat line appeared.

I approached Mrs. Critchley timidly, forced to confront a dead person. Her marble-like face showed a serene mask in death. Her shriveled breasts made me think of her son, how she probably nursed him, as that generation did, and the satisfaction she may have derived from this act of nurturing—an act we men could never emulate or fully grasp the enormity of. Listening to her stilled chest, I heard no heartbeat and no breath sounds. I rechecked her pupils and the blood vessels at the back of her retina and saw death staring back at me. Mrs. Critchley was, indeed, dead. While Fred, my cadaver, had reeked of formaldehyde, Norma Critchley's dead body had no particular smell or odor. The skin over her arms was cold and barely supple and began to mottle with purple blotches.

Sister drew up the sheet to Mrs. Critchley's chin, mumbling what must have been a prayer while placing Mrs. Critchley's rosary in her stiffening hand.

"What do I do now?"

"Sign the death certificate. It's filled in for you. Just write down the time." She added in a reverent voice, "It's lying on my desk," as she pointed in the general direction of her office.

Tearing off my lengthy EKG strip, and rolling it up, I headed to Sister's office. Gazing at the certificate, I saw that Norma Critchley was eighty-nine years old. A few days later, she would have reached her ninetieth birthday. I was struck by the solemnity and finality of her death on this day, the date perhaps predetermined, as stated in the Iliad, "*. . . that death assigned from the day that I was born.*" I had delivered babies, and now, I had witnessed and captured a fellow human's death on my roll of EKG paper.

Raising my voice slightly, I asked, "Sister, where are the cremation papers?" She looked puzzled. "What do you mean?"

"I thought cremation was the norm in the UK. When I was

at the Whittington, all my deceased were cremated. As locum house officer, I received £30 per cremation and the registrar at least £50, you know, ash cash, to encourage cremation and to put the brakes on overcrowded cemeteries."

"Perhaps so," she declared in her sing-song Irish accent, "but the departed Mrs. Critchley is Roman Catholic. They believe in the resurrection of the body after burial, as Jesus Christ was entombed." The family would not want any part of cremation.

Leaving the geriatric ward, I said a silent prayer for Mrs. Critchley. She reminded me so much of my adorable Oma, who had raised me from a bewildered four-year-old to a proud, self-assured German schoolboy.

I felt a sense of calm and wished I had felt this tranquility after my father's death. To comfort those left behind, some say death is our common mystery, and like birth and love, it is a bond that unites us. My father's death certainly didn't have that effect.

An "ah ha" moment occurred to me—that all deaths fall into one of three categories: an electrical event—the muscles and their nerves stop sparking and electrical contractions cease, as with Mrs. Critchley's heart; a nonstop leak in the circulation—continuous bleeding from a wound where all five liters of blood bleed out of the body; and a metabolic event where the cells run out of energy—caused by the higher demands of infections, such as pneumonia and influenza, tuberculosis, malaria, and diphtheria or cancers.

On my way down the stairs, I passed Father George climbing up to give Mrs. Critchley last rites. He greeted me, sounding jovial, unaware that he was too late. When would I next encounter death? Later that night, I would be on call in Casualty.

13

SUICIDE?

It is not possible to know medicine without knowing what a human is.

—Hippocrates

On Monday morning, Dr. Gilliland and I started rounds, with Sister accompanying us. I had admitted Mrs. Kelly at 5 a.m.

"No . . . no. I wasn't trying to commit suicide," the fragile, twenty-seven-year-old had said, adding in a hoarse Irish brogue, "Why would I want to do that when I have two youngsters to care for?"

"You were semi-conscious when they brought you into Casualty early this morning. The nurses and I pumped more than ten white pills out of your stomach. Why did you take so many, and how long have you been taking them?" I asked while Dr. Gilliland observed deferentially.

Sister chimed in, "Your eldest had a nightmare and crawled into your bed. You were out cold. It gave him quite a fright. He called 999." And, after a pause, added, "A lovely boy you have, Mary."

"I had this wicked headache," said Mrs. Kelly, drawing an atypical band of pain around the top of her head. "It kept on getting tighter and tighter. The pain wouldn't go away," and pausing for a moment she added, "so I took more and more pills, wanting it to stop. The past two years, I've had headaches," and as an afterthought, "you know, domestic issues."

It was 2 a.m. when casualty had roused me from a light sleep, stating there was an overdosed patient. While dressing, I formulated a vague plan of action of what I would do.

To my surprise, the charge nurse in casualty was Hanna, who was doing a double shift and had already started an intravenous drip to hydrate Mrs. Kelly. I took my treatment cues from her as she helped talk me through the procedure of inserting a large gastric tube down the patient's throat into the stomach, just like a flight controller talking a novice pilot to a safe landing. A large syringe was attached and the stomach's content was sucked out. Green gastric juices, reeking of vomitus and containing white pills, spilled into an enamel bowl under the patient's chin.

Until the 1960s, most pills in the British pharmacopeia were white. It was a nightmare to identify and distinguish one form of medication from another. However, in Mrs. Kelly's case, identifying the dispensing prescription together with the patient's symptoms gave the night pharmacist the ability to speedily identify that the white pills were codeine compound—codeine with acetaminophen. The codeine depressed breathing, while an excess of acetaminophen would cause liver failure and death. There wasn't an antidote readily available.

As I continued to pump out her stomach, I was relieved to see Mrs. Kelly gradually regain consciousness. When she came around, she looked paler than her pillowcase, with dark rings around her eyes. She complained of dizziness, drowsiness and tachypnea—abnormally rapid, shallow breathing. She lay listless, seemingly heedless of her surroundings, and complaining of a buzzing in her ears from the residual codeine. I examined her and tried to ask a few questions, but she was incoherent—just staring through me. I decided to re-ask Mrs. Kelly the other questions of her overdose later in the morning.

Dawn was breaking over East London when I wrote admitting orders, aware that for the first time in my life, I had the sole responsibility for a patient's life. Hanna looked over my shoulder, checking my orders.

"So, you're new . . . a brand-new doctor," she said with a somewhat playful Irish tone while immodestly looking me over. Despite our surroundings and the strange hour of the day, she was vivacious and flirtatious. Surely, she knew that I was new. Had she not done rounds with me the day before? Yes, I was most certainly a novice at gastric lavage. She had playfully taunted me for my queasiness at the sight of the slopping gastric contents, the accompanying stench, and the coughing and gagging of the patient as she restrained Mrs. Kelly's attempts to pull out the tube that irritated her throat. I ignored her teasing, keen to get some more sleep.

After a quick bath and a hearty English breakfast served in the doctors' common room, by 8 a.m. I was ready for my first ward rounds with Dr. Gilliland and the crew. Sister sat down on the edge of Mrs. Kelly's bed and took her hand.

"And where is Mr. Kelly?"

"He's at sea. You won't tell him, will you, Sister? I just want to get rid of these headaches." She started to cry softly, gripping a soggy tissue. "He left a few weeks ago . . . should be back in six months."

I stared at Mrs. Kelly. What was it about what she said that made me believe her that this wasn't a suicide attempt? I couldn't quite figure it out. But at that moment I thought I did.

I showed the blood work results to Dr. Gilliland. He saw that she had a rare form of anemia caused by extremely low levels of folic acid, unusual for a woman in the reproductive stages of her life. Folic acid is one of the essential B vitamins which the body cannot make, and we get from eating leafy green vegetables. Its function is critical to the production of mature red blood cells. Dr. Gilliland suggested that maybe Mrs. Kelly was not eating sufficient greens. The results also showed that her bone marrow was cranking out immature red cells, reticulocytes, to compensate for the anemia. These immature cells were not efficient oxygen carriers, resulting in low oxygen levels in the blood, causing anemia and her headaches.

Sister, too, had seen the blood results, and tacitly agreed with Dr. Gilliland's suggestion that I might consider asking the dietitian to take Mary's nutrition history to assess vitamin and folic acid intake. As we prepared to move on to the next patient, I wondered about the connection between Mrs. Kelly's results and her headaches. What was the missing link in our knowledge? What was going on in Mrs. Kelly's body? What did we not know?

The dietitian's record showed that Mrs. Kelly was living essentially on bread, butter, and tea. She was eating *some* folate-rich greens, but not enough to meet the minimum daily requirement. Still, a folate deficiency of this magnitude should not have occurred; something else was going on. I was keen to solve this mystery.

Her folic level started to rise toward normal when she ate a balanced hospital diet. We had stopped all her meds because I reasoned that she must be taking something that interfered with folate absorption in the gut. I discussed this possibility with Dr. Gilliland when we did the next rounds. Since her folic level continued to rise toward normal on the hospital diet, no further action was needed. She was concerned about her two small children who were staying with neighbors, she showed no suicidal tendencies, and her headaches had subsided. I discharged her with plans to follow up and review her blood picture when she came back as an outpatient.

On returning two weeks later, she complained of headaches again, and her folic acid level had fallen. "Have you stopped *all* your medications, and are you taking the vitamin supplement?" I asked. She had, but after a pause, she confessed wistfully that since the birth of her last child, she had been taking an oral contraceptive pill. She had started the pill again after we discharged her.

"The pill? Sorry but did I hear you right, Mrs. Kelly? The pill?"

"Yes," she answered.

"That's powerful medicine," I stated, thinking aloud and somewhat irritated, feeling that I had been sideswiped.

"I take it to stop getting pregnant," she said forcefully, then laughed at the delicacy of the moment.

"But your husband is away for six months. Why do you need the pill?" I asked, trying to process all I heard.

She blushed and looked away. There was silence.

Dr. Gilliland reddened.

I wished I could have taken back that question. The naive me was learning fast—she was having an affair, some comfort in her husband's absence.

Her candid confession to me, her physician, revealed my own ambivalent moral stance in the face of loneliness. We become unhinged from everything that anchors us such as our marriage. Just because her husband was not visible in Mary's life didn't diminish her longing for acceptance and the comfort of intimacy—it's the old human story. No matter what, we are alone.

Her answer didn't stop me from becoming curious, but not into her personal make up, background and behavior—that was her life, but to learn if the combined effects of her low dietary folate at home and the added pill were sufficient to cause her anemia.

"Mrs. Kelly, is it possible for you to stop taking the pill for a month?"

She agreed.

At her next outpatient visit, she told me that the headaches were gone. The blood tests showed her folic acid levels had risen and her anemia had improved. Satisfied with hearing these results, she stated she'd start the pill once more.

When a contrite Mrs. Kelly returned at her next follow-up, her folic acid levels had fallen once more, and her headaches had returned, suggesting that the generous levels of the female hormones in the pill were binding the folic acid in her gut.

I had learned at UCH that such deficiency throughout pregnancy is associated with defects in the development of the brain in the fetal stage. According to Dr. Gilliland, the first birth control pills were approved for human use in 1960 and contained a large dose of the two hormones usually produced by the ovaries—estrogen and progesterone.

Making other physicians, particularly obstetricians and family doctors, aware of the hazards of this particular pill was necessary. I wrote up a case history of our findings. As we say in medicine, the THM—the "take-home message"—is that women who took this pill before deciding to have a family may be folic acid deficient at the start their pregnancy. Under such circumstances, physicians should consider giving the woman a folic acid supplement.

It was among the first clinical reports linking high estrogen levels with the binding of folic acid in the gut. The case report interested Dr. Gilliland, who was one of the editors of the *Postgraduate Medical Journal*. We submitted our paper, which was published—my *very first.* In the meantime, a smattering of similar cases began to appear in other British and international medical journals. Consequently, the pill was reformulated, making it safer for women.

When word spread among the nurses that I had cured Mrs. Kelly and solved this vexingly complex medical problem, my status among them was enhanced. An aura of invincibility surrounded me. And with this my self-confidence rose.

Postgraduate Medical Journal (July 1974) 50, 470–472.

Megaloblastic anaemia associated with the oral contraceptive pill

MICHAEL M. MEGUID
M.B., B.S.

WALTER Y. LOEBL
M.R.C.P.

Bethnal Green Hospital, London, E.C.3

Summary

A 27-year-old housewife suffered from severe headaches for a period of 2 years which developed after she started taking an oral contraceptive pill. During this time she gradually developed folic acid deficiency anaemia. This resulted from the inhibition by 'the pill' of the intestinal conjugase system required to deconjugate polyglutamic folate. The patient's headache did not recur after stopping the pill and her anaemia improved with folic acid supplement. The relation between folic acid metabolism and 'the pill' is discussed.

Megaloblastic anaemia associated with oral contraception

A large number of metabolic side effects induced by the contraceptive pill have been described (Drill, 1965). Shojania, Hornady and Barnes (1968), Snyder and Necheles (1969) and Streiff (1970) have described lowered levels of serum folate in women on oral contraceptives, but overt megaloblastic anaemia appears to be uncommon. The following report describes this entirely remediable condition which presented in an insidious form.

I did daily rounds with Sister, occasionally alone with Hanna when she was in charge of the ward, and twice-weekly rounds with Dr. Gilliland and his registrar, Dr. Loebl, who had returned from Israel. We saw our chronic patients and the new ones we had admitted, who I was expected to manage. I was learning new aspects of treating patients every day and was turning my hours of book study into practical knowledge. I was gaining confidence and increasingly viewed with respect.

Among our greatest successes were the weight losses exhibited by the morbidly obese patients. Not only did stoking their metabolism by eating a meal enhance their weight loss, but the addition of a daily exercise program in the physical therapy department helped Mrs. Jenkins become mobile. The exercise programs were initially gentle and, over time, they became more aggressive. This made the patient feel that weight loss was an active form of treatment that was under their control.

We had several other morbidly obese patients during the time I served as Dr. Gilliland's house physician. These patients were discharged in an exultant mood. I was impressed by the amount of weight they lost and also by their claims that their shoe size decreased by one or two fittings and that they looked forward to shopping for new clothes.

Of the original patients I found on the ward when I had first started, Mrs. Sloan, never failed to tell me that she was fine. However, when I did rounds with Drs. Gilliland and Loebl, she recited a litany of complaints, embarrassing and baffling me. One day, Dr. Gilliland turned to me and said, "Take care of this woman," as if I had been ignoring her.

Her rheumatology physician never returned my numerous calls. Mrs. Sloan became my patient. Somewhere in the back of my mind, I remembered a snippet of information from pharmacology that steroids helped patients with rheumatoid arthritis and that a side effect of low dose steroids was a sense of euphoria. When next Dr. Gilliland and the team stood beside Mrs. Sloan and he inquired about her condition, she grinned with a cheerful disposition and said that she was doing much better and was quite satisfied. He turned to me with a wink and said, "Job well done."

Caring for Dr. Silber's geriatric patients was one of the most rewarding and emotionally satisfying tasks I faced. My initial anxieties about the smell of urine and shouts for the nurse were quickly dispelled. I learned much more about the care of the elderly than merely providing a "tune-up." Above all, I got an insight into what lay ahead of me. I was sad to see that some elderly patients never had visitors. I related to the pain of their isolation, loneliness and quiet neglect. I wondered what had happened in their family dynamics that led to this neglect. If only their families cared enough to visit once in a while, their lives would all be enriched. Many were frustrated and sub-clinically depressed because age had robbed them of their everyday abilities. Some recounted loss: people close to them, children who grew up and moved away, spouses and siblings who had died, and friends who began to fade away.

There were a couple of patients who frightened me. Considerably older, they had dementia and were, at times, verbally rambling while at others coherent. Their illness mystified me, for they were physically robust. Near them were two other patients who were clear-headed yet living in bodies that had failed them. Most of the older patients, however, were engaging after I sat with them and showed an interest in their earlier lives—fascinating beyond their often-complex medical problems. Unlike my Oma, who was reticent to talk about her bygone days, some of my geriatric patients were often very willing to open up to reveal their rich pasts—family histories, jobs during the war, and current political opinions. They had all the attributes of any other human: passion, desire, sorrow, regret, grief, anger, and love. Their frailties kept them isolated at home, fearful of going out in case of a fall. Their short stays in the geriatric unit were akin to summer camp. Indeed, some helped about the ward, assisting the tea trolley lady, the librarian, and chatting up the chaplain, if nothing more than for old times' sake.

Riding home on my nights off I reviewed what the day's work had taught me. We were dealing with sick patients, many of whom challenged me. My patients expected me to care for them, alleviate their suffering and make sure they would go home. Like at the rotations where I had trained at University College Hospital, at Bethnal Green I found teamwork among the nurses and doctors was essential. It fostered interdependence among the members of the medical team and respect for the craft each discipline offered. Team leaders like Drs. Gilliland and Silber set the tone of care. They depended on the head nurses and the registrar to perform their duties. As in carrying out the care expected of me by my bosses, as house officers/interns the hospital became my second home. I was proud to be part of the team, to be regarded as essential and dependable, and I instinctively knew that good communication was essential.

I had worked at Bethnal Green Hospital for a couple of months when one evening during dinner, Mrs. Walsh, the older, granny-type woman, asked, "Are you coming to the dance tomorrow evening, luv?" as she poured me a cup of tea. Seeing my baffled look, she added, "Matron arranged a dance for tomorrow night, right here, for the nurses to meet the new doctors."

"I'm off."

"More stew or mash potato, luv?" She was hovering over me as I ate my dinner. "Just come for a few moments, luv, so the young nurses won't be disappointed."

"I'll think about it."

"Matron will be glad to see you. Her girls are far from home and seeking companionship, entertainment and excitement, too." It sounded obligatory.

The next evening on my way home, I popped into the dance and stood at the door. The furniture was cleared to one side and the room was filled with a seething mass of men and women who danced frantically to the Beatles refrain "I want to hold your hand" that blared from a speaker in the poorly lit, smoke-filled dining room. Flesh, alive, throbbing music, unheard urgent ER pagers, flowing alcohol, moving to Marion Faithfull's hypnotizing slow dances, the sweaty clinging bodies coupled—for better or worse—for one night or longer.

Matron smiled at me and offered a glass of ale drawn from a keg. I stepped into the room, watching the dancing couples, barely recognizing the nurses out of uniform. The ratio of nurses to doctors was probably four to one. I looked across the room and saw Hanna wearing a white blouse and a pencil skirt and dancing with one of the other house physicians at the hospital. When the music stopped, she weaved her way over to me. "You came, that's nice," she beamed at me over the noisy crowd. Her hair, with a loose fringe, framed her smiling face while her eyes twinkled mischievously.

With the start of the next fast song, we danced, face to face, side by side, bumping into other couples in the crowded room. She rocked in front of me full of life and swirled her hips with the beat, twirling around and about—her body language provocative. I liked it. Victoria would never let herself dance so freely.

She sang out loud with Paul and John with wanton abandon, obviously enjoying herself. The slower "Hey Jude" followed. She grabbed my hand and drew me into her orbit; the aura of her perfume stirred some lusty thoughts.

"Come and join us at the pub after the dance," she ventured between songs.

"I've got to go home. My wife is waiting for me."

On the Tube, I joined the evening rush hour crowds crammed into the speeding carriages under London. I had done my duty as a responsible physician to the Matron and the community of nurses at Bethnal Green. I tried to get in touch with my agitated feelings, which were somewhat aroused and made me feel uncomfortable. I raised my hand to my nose, revisiting the scent that Hanna had left on me. I couldn't wait for Victoria to come home. I wanted her.

Darkness had descended by the time I reached our warm but empty flat. Victoria was late in coming home. It was comforting to feel her warm body next to me when we finally tumbled into bed.

14

THE PROPINQUITY OF LONELINESS

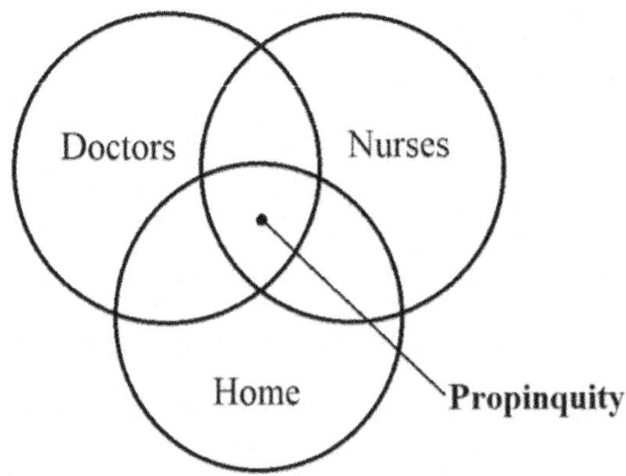

The most terrible poverty is loneliness, and the feeling of being unloved.

—Mother Teresa

In October of 1968, dusk was settling over Bethnal Green early. The neighborhood pubs had just opened when I stepped into the street, heading home midway through my six-month stint. Four nurses in their uniforms and capes paused to enter the Dundee Arms. Hanna, taller and slimmer than her three companions, spotted me. We locked eyes for a brief moment and she beckoned me to join them. I hesitated, then waved politely and turned away, heading down Cambridge Heath Road to the Tube station. I wasn't much of a drinker and not good at small talk. What would we talk about? Would the conversation degrade to medical jokes and forced laughter to show that we were human, equals in the absence of a medical hierarchy?

A one-on-one situation I could manage. Hanna was intriguing and alluring. I was captivated by the intensity of her glance, her boldness, her playfulness and the seductive intonations of her Irish accent that resonated in my head. Her attention flattered me. These feelings, though, unsettled me.

Our flat was dark when I arrived home, and the place had a cold, empty feeling to it—not like the warm pub I had passed up. I looked about for something to eat in the glaring light of the kitchenette. The cupboards were barren, apart from some staples and bread. Neither Victoria nor I had had time to go grocery shopping. In the tiny refrigerator, I found some cheese and eggs. I expected Victoria to arrive home at any moment. I wanted to embrace her, to ground me again. If she hadn't eaten, maybe we'd make cheese omelets. If she wasn't too tired, we could go for curry at our favorite Indian restaurant, the Agra in Whitfield Street near UCH, where I knew the proprietor, Mr. Subhan Sultan.

During the homeward journey, the urgency and energy that fueled my day had gradually drained and my whole body was weary. I made a pot of tea and poured myself a cup and listened to the 6 p.m. BBC radio news. Exhausted, I plonked down in our only armchair, looked through our mail, and flicked through the *British Medical Journal.* Nothing of interest.

I wondered, should I have joined the nurses and ordered a plate of piping hot Shepherd's pie or steak and kidney pudding? Outside, the evening rush hour was at its apogee. The noise of cars and buses flashed by our closed window, occasionally rattling them. Buses filled with office-weary passengers headed north along Albany Street toward Camden Town or St. John's Woods, and others headed into central London, carrying early revelers, perhaps into the theater district or to fancy restaurants.

I stared across the dimly lit room through the lace curtains at the passing dark shadows. With each bus that halted outside the house, I imagined Victoria alighting, raising my spirits. I anticipated the brief ring of the doorbell, announcing her arrival, her key in the lock and her footfall on the stairs.

None came.

Not this bus.

Maybe the next.

With each disappointment, the insecurity of my loneliness rose and exponentially grew—a frightening feeling. Night's darkness invaded the room—a dark blackness that I could not keep out, engulfing the atmosphere, overwhelming my mood and persisting like an internal demon even after I drew the curtain. I was annoyed with myself for the despair of not having come to terms with my old "abandonment trauma." No matter how much I argued with myself about the absurdity of these ferocious torments or tried to soothe myself, the dark fears marinated torments of loneliness in me. When I felt secure, contented with life and in Victoria's sheltering presence, the festering sore of the past appeared to have healed.

Where was Victoria? Had something happened to her? I wanted her home, even though I knew her work as a medical student was demanding and that she was preoccupied. I loved seeing her. It was so reassuring. I admired her face and figure. I loved listening to her idle chatter of the mundane news about our friends, the goings-on in the hospital, her medical achievements and frustrations of the day and telling her about mine. The minute she walked into our safe nest, our little abode, the gripping void of darkness would vanish, and I would be cured for that moment.

Hanna's smile, her striking blond hair and her uncanny resemblance to Julie Christie in *Dr. Zhivago* started to encroah into my pit of despair. I brushed it away. But like the Raven in Poe's poem, Hanna kept intruding into my thoughts. If I had joined the nurses in the pub, what harm would have been done? It would be comforting to have their company. What if we met on the evenings that I was wretched because my beloved Victoria wouldn't be home? I imagined that I could manage a plutonic friendship. The thought consoled me as I drifted to sleep on our double bed, waiting for her, for my Victoria.

Then, I saw Victoria through the coffin lid. She was standing with mourners around the pit's edge, her delicate fingers holding a bouquet of white lilies. A thin veil partially hid her face. Yet I saw her eyes, those striking eyes that had caught my attention when I first saw her, now bright and cheery, her lips moving with the vicar's recitation "*. . . till thou return unto the ground for out of it wast thou taken for dust thou art, and unto dust shalt thou return . . .*" As my coffin descended into darkness the intense light from the pit's head diminished as it became smaller. The lilies and earth crashed on the coffin's lid.

I yelled, "No, no I don't want to die. I want to live. I want to feel alive, not to be parted from you." And as I struggled to get out, my arms knocked over the glass of water by the bedside and I awoke, unable to distinguish water from sweat on my face.

I rose. It was well past 8 p.m. I washed my face, brushed my teeth, and wished she'd be home. Drifting into a pre-slumber haze, I wondered if I was more attuned to Hanna's unbridled vivre and joy in life. Was Victoria's personality a good fit for mine? What a terrible question. Before I could sort out these nebulous thoughts, I once more fell into a deep sleep, aware when Victoria plunked in next to me. I wish I had bucked up the courage to tell her that on nights like this, I missed and longed for her dearly. But more importantly, I wanted to tell her that my life was incomplete without her.

A few days later, I learned that Hanna was in charge of the ward during the night shift. I tried to fall asleep in my on-call room but couldn't stop thinking about the way she looked at me with admiration. Like an addict, I was drawn to her. As I crept through the dim ward at 2 a.m., my heart pounded, and I hoped she'd be the only nurse I'd encounter. Her scent drew me closer until her image emerged among the beds.

"What are you doing here?" her Irish voice sang out through the darkness as she approached me.

"I couldn't sleep. Eh, just checking on my patients." The buckle of her red belt caught the dim light. Even in her nurses uniform she looked stunning. Her starched pinafore exaggerated the outline of her breasts. Her smile was tender and welcoming. I gazed at her.

"Are you a night owl?"

"No, actually, I'm an early morning person—you know, the surgical type, compulsive and obsessive."

"It's quiet and I have a break coming up. Cup of tea?"

"I'd love one. Not too strong so it won't keep me awake."

She boiled the water as I settled in a chair opposite her in Sister's office. We were alone. The thrill of temptation trickled down my spine. I watched her every move, delighting in her presence, wondering how old she was. Perhaps twenty-three.

"You don't need sugar. You're sweet enough," she chuckled as I stirred a spoonful into my cup. "So, which patient kept you awake?" she teased.

I smiled, slightly embarrassed at her recognizing my ploy.

"Where in Ireland are you from?"

"County Tyrone. You know, Northern Ireland. From a farm in Richhill. It's just south of Belfast."

"Well, I'm from Cairo. Born with camel dung between my toes."

She chuckled. "You don't say . . . Egypt." She dragged the word out, amused. "I've never been there."

"I've never been to Ireland."

Standing up, she said, "Well, let's go. I can show you around. The bushes are lush and green," and seeing me mischievously raise one eyebrow at the word bush, she blushed and completed her sentence, "not dull and gray like here."

"Would the rose garden in Regent's Park do?" I said playfully.

I had convinced myself that my friendship with Hanna would be platonic. The Park was a neutral place. We met on a Saturday afternoon at the Regent's Bar and Kitchen Café. It was an overcast day with the sun peeking through the clouds. I arrived early, heart in my mouth, and watched her approach. She looked delightful. I was flattered that she had agreed to meet me and looked forward to getting to know her.

I wondered if anyone we knew would see us. Unease and guilt accompanied me as we walked about, ambling between strollers. I managed to silence the alarm bells ringing in my brain telling myself I could keep matters under control. Hanna didn't want any tea but went for a McVitie's Penguin, loving the milk chocolate-covered crunchy biscuit. I had one too. As we walked, I did most of the talking—nervous chatter about myself—even though I was curious about her, her past, her dreams, her aspirations. Did she have family here or connections that attracted her to England, like so many Irish? I did not ask, and she did not offer an inlet into her life.

The skies opened up and we got soaked as we huddled with other ramblers under a meager canopy. Unsure of what to do or where to go, I nervously suggested John Rackey's nearby flat. He was in Florida and had given me the key to pop in from time to time to water his only plant and pick up the mail. We could dry off, have a cup of tea, and chat. Could we? I sensed I was driving over a cliff with no brakes. The thought of being alone with her frightened me. I worried because the other me, the me who was lonely, the fucking foreigner who found consolation in the warmth of a woman's body, might win out. The flat was too intimate a setting. I regretted making the offer.

John's flat, number 212, was dim and airless as we hesitantly crept into the small foyer, reluctant to switch on the light. We whispered as if not wishing to disturb an occupant, a forgotten cat, or the neighbors. What would John say if he knew I had brought a girl here? I could almost hear his retort, "The road to hell is paved with good intentions," he'd say, two index fingers on his forehead, mimicking the devil's horns.

We removed our wet coats and soaking shoes in the small kitchenette. We could barely move about without bumping into each other. Under her dripping M&S coat, now hanging over the kitchen chair, Hanna wore a red blouse and a stylish beige chamois skirt. Despite the times we had been together during rounds, I only now noticed that she was about my height, tall for a woman, and voluptuous. The erotic tension became palpable as she stood opposite me drying her hair on the single kitchen towel.

There was only one chair in the breakfast area, off that a toilet with a bath, and a single bed set in a dim alcove. I didn't find a teapot, only an electric kettle. There was a tin of Nescafé and one labeled hot chocolate. No milk. Ah yes, John drank only coffee. Hanna refused my offer to make her a cup.

We perched on the edge of John's bed, chatting. Hanna repeatedly tugged on her short skirt, which kept riding up her stockinged thighs.

"Sister McGrady told me that you didn't trust her when she told you one of her patients was dying."

"Of course, I trusted her. Why would she be talking about me to you?"

"We were at supper in the nurses' dorm and chatting about the new house officers."

"Ah! Gossiping. And what did she say?"

"She likes you. You're smart." After hesitating, she added, "The best looking of the three house officers." I blushed. "Did she tell you about the O-sign and Q-sign that go with death?"

"You're having me on. The O- and Q-signs? Tell me."

"Well, you're walking down the ward and you find an old person in bed with their mouth open and their lips making an O. When you go over to them, they are dead." She imitated a perfect O with her lips and laughed. She looked charmingly funny.

"What about the Q?" I asked, engaging in her playfulness.

"That's when their tongue sticks out to one side," she said, chuckling after mimicking it. Her perfect teeth and the sight of her protruding tongue aroused me in the increasingly sexual atmosphere. Our proximity brought me into her body aura, mixed with a perfume that aroused me further. I restrained myself from impulsively kissing her—I heard the alarm bell signaling danger.

I hated being with her. I regretted even arranging our rendezvous. What would I do if we crossed that fidelity barrier? Secrecy, lies and gnawing guilt would follow. Who else would know? I loathed myself. I should just get up and leave.

The sensual tension was too great to walk back. In the close confines of the alcove Eros prevailed. I kissed her lips tentatively, tasting her strawberry gloss, fearful she would reject me. Assured that she welcomed my advances, we kissed more ferociously and fell back onto John's bedspread.

"I mustn't get this skirt too rumpled or stained," she whispered, "I borrowed it from another nurse."

"It looks nice," I said, wondering what she meant by "stained." As I watched, she stood up and unabashedly peeled it off, revealing a skimpy, laced white panty.

A mix of emotions swirled through me as she descended the escalator at Great Portland Street to take the Circle Line back to Bethnal Green. I felt relieved that it was over. And it seemed that no one among the evening crowd had recognized us together. The tension and anxiety of the situation left me with a monumental headache. I felt guilty. I had done something utterly wrong, yet thrilling. The exhilaration of being together came from reliving the intense sensation of my first sexual encounter in Manchester, my seduction by a new widow in Hamburg while waiting for her husband's body to arrive from Nairobi, my fantasy of Julie Christie, and the feeling of a stranger wanting me, accepting me, and loving me. Yet I felt a mixture of repugnance and shame. Thank God this was done with.

It troubled me that Hanna was very comfortable with our encounter. I wished that she wasn't, so as to put the brakes on this event. There was no hesitation on her part, no awkwardness or shyness. It was so different from being with Victoria, whose shyness repressed me from beholding what I longed to see of her body and which aroused my ardor. Hanna was easygoing with her body and with mine, not to mention with acts of intimacy—new ones unfamiliar to me and surprising. Was she part of the 60s' sexual liberation movement? A good Catholic girl from Ireland?

The thought added to the thrill. Where had she gained this experience? I wasn't the first. An inner voice said *why should you be?* She was in her twenties, young, smart, good-looking, and ambitious. Having been raised on a farm, she no doubt saw animals in heat.

How could I see her on the ward and pretend nothing had happened between us? I knew what she hid beneath her nurse's uniform and the transformation in her persona when we were together. She turned me on. At the same time, I wondered if I was into more than I could handle?

Victoria wasn't home. Feeling like a sullied dog, I had a quick bath. Drying myself off, I wondered if Hanna was thinking of me? Was she quietly joyful at her conquest?

There were more clandestine meetings. I sensed Hanna may have said something about me among her circle of close friends—Irish nurses living in the nursing school dorm—because she came wearing borrowed clothing and shoes.

I perceived the vibes from other nurses during the workday, the young ones cheery and hopeful, with an air of informality and awareness; the older or senior nurses, once friendly enough, now responded with a hint of some reservation, misgivings, and even disdain. Was I imagining all this? Anyway, I'd soon be leaving Bethnal Green.

When I was with Victoria, anxiety and shame about Hanna shadowed me. Did she suspect? Could rumors have reached her? Had I accidentally mentioned Hanna's name in my sleep for I was known to talk in my sleep? The only time I was emotionally free of the worries and deception, of the other me, was when Victoria and I went for the weekend to our Isle of Serenity—in the Solent.

As we trained down together, my burden of remorse and dishonor lightened with each mile from London. The relief was overwhelming. Alone with my wife once more, we traveled into a past where we had loved so freely, so enjoyably. It was at such times I strongly felt that my dallying had to stop. "Yes, this must stop," I whispered to myself when I was alone, stewing in my regret. I made this promise on more than one occasion, but like the many other promises that my patients made to quit smoking, to stop drinking, or to lose a few pounds, the draw of the forbidden was too great.

Approaching the end of my six-month appointment, I received a brief note from Dr. Gilliland. He wanted to see me.

Terror gripped me. Had he heard a rumor about Hanna and me? Or worse, had he seen us together in London? Was he going to admonish me, just as Mother had when I was four? I wanted to retch.

What would be my defense? Was it that I was alone so much because my wife was too occupied with her studies to love me? No. I couldn't say that—it was a cop-out. Besides, it wasn't Victoria's fault. Perhaps he would be more understanding if I said I found Hanna attractive, always available, and that we enjoyed each other's company. Or with a light laugh and a wink, I might say, "She is a fantastic kisser and good in bed, you know." To reassure him, I'd say that it would end when I moved on to my surgical house job. I was sure it would.

Dr. Gilliland's concern was about my next appointment. "Have you given any thought to where you want to do your house surgeon's rotation?"

My pounding heart and shallow breathing slowed. "I'm still interested in doing it at UCH," I said, still fearful he might raise the other matter.

"I hear that Mr. Milling, Mr. Kingdom and Mr. Archer are

looking for someone who also has an academic bent. Some surgeons on his team are doing an interesting study in women with certain types of breast cancer." Pointing to just below his eyebrow he continued, "They are going in through the nose and the sphenoid sinus to remove the pituitary in women with advanced breast cancer." The pituitary is the master endocrine gland located in the brain; it stimulates the hormone production of the other glands in the body. "The hope is that removing it will reduce the size of metastatic tumors that have spread from the breast to different parts of the body. Would that appeal to you?"

He continued, "It wouldn't be general surgery. But he and his team are very successful."

I hesitated. Head and neck surgery? As if to reassure me he said, "Not general surgery, but cutting-edge surgery for sure. And related to breast disease, which you mentioned is becoming more attractive."

"Thank you for thinking of me. Yes. I'll apply."

"Well, good luck. I think it's a good fit, and you'd get back to UCH, away from here." I sensed that Dr. Gilliland was a sensitive person, and that he was an epitome of discretion if, indeed, he was aware of the situation.

As we rose, he hesitated. "Your name came up during a conversation with Rosenheim," he said quietly. I froze.

"I mentioned your stellar performance and your observation about folic acid. I'm glad you're writing that up—it's really quite important."

What was coming next? "He's a strange fellow, really. You know, we briefly crossed paths in Palestine. I think he stayed to fight for the new State of Israel."

It took me a while to digest the implication of what he said.

Three years later Dr. Gilliland, Victoria and I had dinner together.

PART III

LONDON

WINTER 1968 TO SUMMER 1969

We all love ourselves more than other people,
but care more about their opinion than our own.
—Marcus Aurelius

15

MY OWN OPERATING LIST

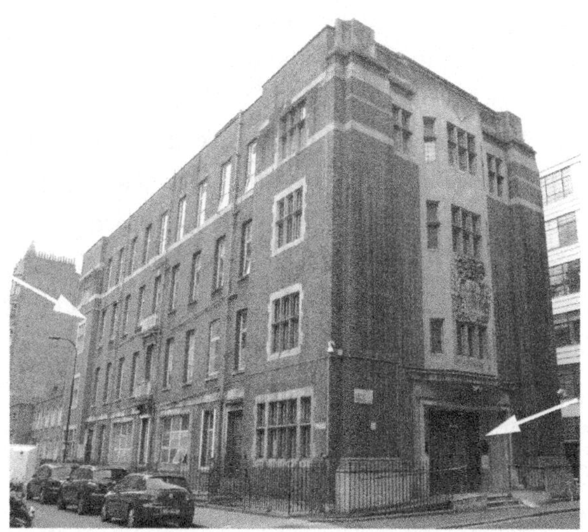

Royal Ear Hospital, Philafrenzy, CC BY-SA 4.0, via Wikimedia Commons. Arrow on left is the hospital, and on right is the House Officers' quarters connected by underground tunnels to each other and UCH.

Only those who risk going too far can possibly find out how far one can go. —T. S. Eliot

Mr. Kingdom, the consultant surgeon, interviewed me for the house officer job at the end of his busy outpatient clinic at Huntly Street. We sat in the white-tiled waiting area with its high set windows after the nurses had left for the day. We had met three years previously when I had several episodes of severe tonsillitis. He relaxed in his tweed jacket and flannel trousers and looked more in need of a late afternoon drink than to sit there quizzing me.

The Royal Ear Hospital was founded in 1816 as the Dispensary for Diseases of the Ear. As the need for space and operating facilities grew, the hospital ultimately was built in Huntly Street and became part of University College Hospital. Although physically separate, Casualty, the hospital, the physician's residence and the nursing home were connected via common underground tunnels to the Royal Ear Hospital, where I now sat with Mr. Kingdom.

Like in Professor Rosenheim's case, I was the only candidate, but unlike that odious situation, Mr. Kingdom was alone and didn't have my student records in front of him. I didn't anticipate an abusive interview but I was ready for anything that was going to be thrown at me. Although I didn't know much about ear, nose and throat, or even head and neck cancers or their surgery, I had done a reasonable job as locum house surgeon on Professor Pilcher's unit, even overcoming my differences with Mr. Hart, and felt more secure as a surgical candidate for Mr. Kingdom's House Surgeon's job.

We faced each other in straight-back wooden chairs. "Your references are top drawer." I felt a deep wave of pleasant satisfaction. He continued, "The job starts in two weeks, and I think you'll like being back at UCH. Very civilized place," adding, "well, you know all about it." He was right; I was keen to be back, although the two-week delay was unexpected.

He mentioned the two other senior consultants who operated at the Royal Ear Hospital and went on to briefly mention the registrars with whom I'd work—a senior one from New Zealand and one from Trinidad, who was doing a maxillofacial fellowship. "We have an interesting mix of cases, you know, the bread-and-butter stuff like tonsillectomies, mastoid and sinus drainage. Also, the usual mix of tumors." He hesitated, expecting a response. I merely nodded. "Cancers of the tongue and larynges, and head and neck in general. I hear you're interested in surgery. We will arrange for you to have your own operating list of three to four cases that you can do on a Saturday morning. The lads will help you. That's a great leap toward becoming a surgeon. My focus deals with hearing loss due to tumors and, of course, from the three bones of the inner ear." I listened carefully.

Accepting this job would bring me back into the academic world, broaden my surgical experience, and aid in the prospects of my future surgical career. Above all, I would be having my own patients to operate on! It wasn't the exact surgical appointment I had wished for, preferring abdominal surgery, but perhaps I might even enjoy operating in the head and neck domain.

He looked at me, trying to weigh-up my reactions, for I'd said little—in reality, what was there to say? Raising his voice, he said, "I did a stapedectomy, you know, removing one of the bones in the middle ear on a middle-aged woman for hearing loss." I nodded my understanding and he continued. "When she came back for follow-up, I asked her if her hearing had improved. 'Oh, it's marvelous,' she raved, 'and it's a good contraceptive. Before the operation, when my husband and I went to bed he'd say, 'Are you tired or what?' And I'd reply, 'What'" Mr. Kingdom roared with laughter as he rose and shook my hand. "I look forward to working with you. I'll see you soon. Have a well-deserved break."

16

AN UNSETTLING STATISTIC

Lies, damn lies and statistics.
—Benjamin Disraeli

It was a strange feeling to be free for two weeks. I was accustomed to having every minute of a twenty-four-hour day filled with patient-related activities, including disturbed nights and work-filled weekends. My sudden freedom left me feeling apprehensive. What should I be doing right now? What was I missing? Was I late for rounds or a meeting with social services? Had I fallen asleep from fatigue and forgotten the telephone call about a patient in Casualty?

Reading most of the news columns on each page of the daily *Times* occupied part of what seemed like an endless day. With Victoria gone much of the time, the house was silent. I could hear the ceaseless ticking of our carriage clock on the mantle resonating through our small flat. Victoria had made our home comfortable, and the furniture we had borrowed from her mother and grandmother added to our secure world. Shopping and preparing an evening meal for my tired wife only took up a fraction of my time. I loved going to our local Tesco supermarket and striking up conversations with strangers and shop clerks to recapture simple human contact. It validated me. I bought Victoria flowers. They added so much joy to our domain. I put up a notice at the medical school seeking a squash partner and, indeed, found one to play with.

Although I was lonely, I resisted the temptation to contact Hanna, even though, at times, I'd daydream of her. She would never know of my occasional longing, my random fantasy of us together. I was certain that she would never suspect my aching for her and that she had moved on with her life, where I had been a transient, an insignificant diversion.

One morning, my doorbell rang. A youngish woman in a wool coat who was holding a clipboard stood there, gazing up at me.

"Hello. I'm from the Ministry of Social Security. Are you currently working?"

"No."

"Are you employed?"

"No."

"So, you are unemployed." Before I could process her statement, she continued, "Well, you must go to the unemployment office in Marylebone and register. They will help you find another job."

"But I'm a physician; I have a job lined up in ten days."

"Are you sticking your social security contribution stamps each week?"

"No."

"Well then, until you start a new job, please go to the unemployment office to register and collect your benefits." With that, she left.

Shocked, I suddenly realized I had become a statistic—one of the nation's jobless. This officious woman could not see that I was a doctor. The very thought of being unemployed, the very label of going on the dole rocked me—implying poverty and dismissing my years of striving, the hard-earned title I had achieved and my standing in society as a physician.

I felt irritated at her intrusion into my life and confused as well. How did I get my self-worth from external validation? What would I tell Victoria? She was heavily involved and preoccupied with her studies, and my two weeks of being out of work, idle, redundant, and then being told to receive benefits was embarrassing shameful.

Uncomfortable and conspicuous in my usual suit and tie, I stood in the queue that snaked silently about itself and led to the teller at its head. There were few conversations among the group. I felt acutely embarrassed to be standing with house painters in their paint-covered overalls, carrying paint pots and brushes, and plumbers with their toolkits, mainly men, who were apparently jobless. Were these the individuals I read about who were abusing the social welfare system? Or truly out of a job? Now I was joining them.

I was a respectable physician, a surgeon no less, with integrity and the prospect of work in a few days. Collecting unemployment made me uncomfortable. I felt I was a fraud—ripping off social services. Despite these anxious feelings, I was also pleased at milling about with other humans and overhearing their occasional prosaic murmurs. We stood in the queue, each man with his own reason. Did they also feel that their dignity, their professionalism, was stained or defiled by standing in this line? I couldn't tell.

I tried to explain my situation to the clerk, who listened patiently and then resumed asking me questions. She filled in my answers on a form. Finally, she said that the system would stick the weekly twenty-four shillings and ten pence unemployment stamp on my behalf and that I should expect six pounds and change in my post office Girocheck account. With that, I walked out into the mid-day sunlight, leaving the humiliating feelings behind.

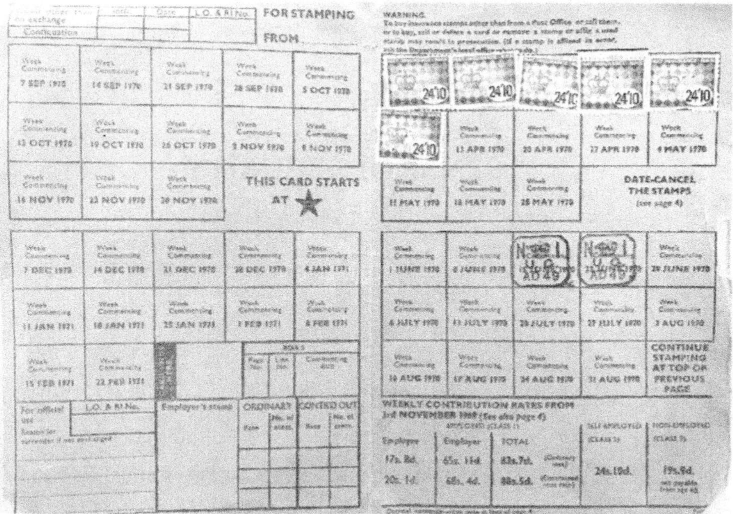

FOR STAMPING FROM

Week Commencing	Week Commencing	Week Commencing	Week Commencing	Week Commencing
7 SEP 1970	14 SEP 1970	21 SEP 1970	28 SEP 1970	5 OCT 1970
12 OCT 1970	19 OCT 1970	26 OCT 1970	2 NOV 1970	9 NOV 1970
16 NOV 1970	23 NOV 1970	30 NOV 1970	THIS CARD STARTS AT ★	
7 DEC 1970	14 DEC 1970	21 DEC 1970	28 DEC 1970	4 JAN 1971
11 JAN 1971	18 JAN 1971	25 JAN 1971	1 FEB 1971	8 FEB 1971
15 FEB 1971	22 FEB 1971			

For official use — L.O. & RI No. — Employer's stamp — ORDINARY — CONTRACTED OUT

WARNING

24'10	24'10	24'10	24'10	24'10
24'10	Week Commencing 13 APR 1970	Week Commencing 20 APR 1970	Week Commencing 27 APR 1970	Week Commencing 4 MAY 1970
Week Commencing 11 MAY 1970	Week Commencing 18 MAY 1970	Week Commencing 25 MAY 1970	DATE-CANCEL THE STAMPS (see page 4)	
Week Commencing 1 JUNE 1970	Week Commencing 8 JUNE 1970			Week Commencing 29 JUNE 1970
Week Commencing 6 JULY 1970	Week Commencing 13 JULY 1970	Week Commencing 20 JULY 1970	Week Commencing 27 JULY 1970	Week Commencing 3 AUG 1970
Week Commencing 10 AUG 1970	Week Commencing 17 AUG 1970	Week Commencing 24 AUG 1970	Week Commencing 31 AUG 1970	CONTINUE STAMPING AT TOP OF PREVIOUS PAGE

WEEKLY CONTRIBUTION RATES FROM 3rd NOVEMBER 1969 (See also page 4)

Employee	Employer	TOTAL	SELF-EMPLOYED (CLASS 2)	NON-EMPLOYED (CLASS 3)
17s. 8d.	65s. 11d.	83s.7d.	24s.10d.	19s.9d.
20s. 1d.	68s. 4d.	88s.5d.		

When Victoria came home that evening, she shrugged off the news of my statistical label, pleased that I was home, this night and every night for the next fortnight. At the end of the first week, we had an exotic meal at the Agra, attentively fussed over by Mr. Subhan Sultan, who brought out specialty dishes, samples of the Indian wedding banquet that was going on a floor above us. We wandered home, hand in hand, and fell into our bed together. Exhausted by our caresses and loving, she fell asleep, our torsos partially entwined, hers uncovered. Moonlight bounced off her smooth curves that resembled the shining white marble of a Michelangelo.

17

A SENSE OF SECURITY

He felt now that he was not simply close to her
but that he did not know where he ended and she began.
—Leo Tolstoy

The relief of moving back into UCH's house officers' quarters on University Street shook off the unhappy countenance of unemployment as I again took on a mantle of dignity: the title of House Surgeon. Meals were served each day in the house officers' quarters some distance away via the underground tunnel.

Mr. Kingdom and the other consultants operated three times a week; two days were for seeing outpatients. Eight to twelve patients arrived after 2 p.m. on the day before surgery. Depending on their diagnoses, it took me between four and six hours in the afternoon and early evening to see all the new patients, during which time I worked closely with the charge nurse. My responsibilities included clerking them and getting their X-rays from the main hospital via the tunnels, getting consent forms signed, explaining their operation, and generally preparing them for the next day's procedure.

After I had dinner, served in the physician's quarters at eight, I attended to the postoperative care of the day's cases. In the very late evenings, I'd read about the various ailments of head and neck pathology, their disease processes, and the operations to be performed the next day.

On the nights when I was on call and Victoria was free, she would join me to be together—creeping up the back stairs behind the beadle's back.

"Oh, it's great to see you," I said, wrapping her in my arms.

She kicked off her shoes, "I'm exhausted. I had a long day. Tedious pathology lectures given by a poor speaker. My notes are awful."

I held her at arm's length and looked into her tired eyes. "Sorry, sweetheart. Use my *Lecture Notes on Pathology* by Cotton. It's good. I think it's in the stack of books on the floor." I added, "It's a bit marked up, but clearly written."

"I'm just drained. It's been a long day."

"But you look wonderful."

"My hair's a mess. I didn't get to wash it this morning."

"Have you eaten? Had dinner?"

"Sort of. I'm fine. I didn't have time to change."

"How's Shirley?"

"The same. She's coming up from the Island to see her therapist, and wants to see Granny in Petersfield, too, on her way here. She mentioned lunch with me."

"That's nice. Where?"

"I just can't. I'd love to, but I have lectures and I'm on a busy service." She paused, sitting on the edge of the bed.

"Staying or would you sleep better at home?"

"I'll stay but I have to pee. Check the way is clear," she said as I opened the door. I loved having her with me. Her mere presence made me feel whole. In her arms I fell into a deep and pure sleep—the peaceful slumber of restorative sleep needed by a surgeon—an antidote to stress.

During the week, she'd sneak out in the early hours of the morning. On weekends when I was on call, I had to get up early to do rounds. She seldom slept late, not wanting to lie alone in my room. Such was our life.

After a while, I felt like a lackey. I was working on the wards in a different world from the surgeons who were having fun in the operating theater dealing with complex operations for cancer of the throat or the larynx. I didn't see them for long stretches during the day. Did they know I even existed? When they finished a case, they'd accompany their patient onto the ward and give instructions to Sister or the charge nurse and me about their patient's post-operative care and then disappear.

When I complained to my friendly, understanding Afro-Trinidadian Maxillofacial Fellow, Desmond, he recognized my frustration. He started to take some of the slack by clerking a few of the admitted patients when he was between cases, freeing me to go to the outpatient clinic to see patients with Mr. Kingdom. I seldom saw the senior registrar, Mr. Knight, and began to wonder if indeed he worked at UCH.

Desmond was a cheerful man with a ready smile and a baritone voice. I was charmed by his attitude toward life, his Caribbean accent, and his love for different ethnic foods. On more than a couple of occasions when we were on call together or he had operated late into the day, we went to the Agra for a late dinner. He was easygoing, friendly and quick to laugh, telling me about his life with his grandmother in Trinidad who had raised him. He resurrected my reminiscences of my Oma who became my surrogate mother after my mother dumped me in post-war Wedel and disappeared from my life. Desmond didn't tell me outright what happened to his mother, but from hints he dropped here and there throughout our friendship, I surmised she had left him after the war to work in England. His chatter also reminded me of the warm breeze and azure Caribbean waters, the Antiguan beach sand between my toes and the vision of Victoria lying on a red beach towel sunning herself.

We chatted about the trajectory of a surgeon's training, the peculiarities of each consultant and what we knew of their personal lives. Eventually, the conversation came around to bigotry. He had encountered similar narrow-mindedness and refutations to my experiences when he came to England, but his tolerance of such prejudices was better. As a man of color, he chuckled, "If they had not come to us and impoverished us centuries ago, we wouldn't be over here." Leaning back in his chair he roared with laughter. There was an element of truth in what he said.

Our common bonds were the pain of the rejection that we had encountered, the unsettling questioning of identity and our eagerness to operate. He got his share of cutting, particularly on head and neck cancer operations. I had not and was hungry to cut. I related Mr. Kingdom's promise to 'arrange for you to have your own operating list of three to four cases that you can do on a Saturday morning.' Desmond organized for the admissions of patients from the waiting list and on Friday I enthusiastically admitted them.

Peter was a seventeen-year-old boy who presented with a midline neck swelling above the thyroid, which had become more prominent in the past few months as it grew to a one-inch mass. It was painless, round, smooth, soft, and moved up and down when he swallowed and when he protruded his tongue. When I shone a light on it from a pen torch, the mass was translucent, indicating that it was a thyroglossal cyst.

I had learned of these cysts during embryology classes at University College. The anatomy prosectors had been right when they told us that the basic sciences would become useful when we became physicians. At that time, it was hard to believe them. During development, the thyroid gland migrates from the back of the tongue down into the neck to its adult position. Usually, the track closes after the migration. Occasionally, remnants get hung up along the route and develop into a thyroglossal cyst during early adulthood. Its removal prevents the unsightly cyst from becoming infected.

After Peter was anesthetized the following morning, the circulating nurse washed his neck with an antiseptic solution and covered the surrounding area with sterile towels. Desmond gave me the scalpel, and with a nod from the anesthetist, who had finished injecting an antibiotic, I made a three-inch horizontal skin incision through the underlying subcutaneous tissue and the thin sheet of neck muscle, the platysma. Desmond held the skin edges apart, electrocoagulated the bleeders and sucked out the little pools of blood. The bulging cyst peeked out well above the hyoid bone, between the strap muscles of the neck. I dissected the cyst out from the surrounding tissue and cut it out from the shriveled fibrous tract. Desmond irrigated the tissue debris with saline, and then I closed the wound, placing a small drain that would remove any extra fluid or blood that would accumulate in the dead space. I would see Peter afterward in the ward.

My next patient was moved into the operating room. I had clerked and examined Susan, a nineteen-year-old art student. She was suffering from repeated tonsillitis, and her tonsils were flaming red golf balls with little clusters of pus in their crypts. The tonsils are lymph glands that nestle in a bed between two muscular pillars—part of the throat or pharyngeal muscle group at the back of the mouth. They fight attacks of viral or bacterial infections that enter the nose and mouth. After repeated inflammations, they become enlarged, chronically disease ridden and a source of poisoning that could lead to heart valve damage later in life. Susan's needed removing.

Victoria's and mine had been removed by Mr. Kingdom three years previously. When I awoke from anesthesia, my throat was on fire with pain. Excruciating electric shocks raced throughout my neck and head. Swallowing caused howling discomfort and instant regret that I had agreed to the operation. The pain had a musical quality, like nails scratching down a blackboard. The only pain med offered was soluble aspirin, which I had to swallow. This act alone had the high-pitched squeaking of tram wheels taking a curve in Cairo. By day seven, the pain had become bearable, allowing me to transition from ice cream and popsicles to soft food. I could hardly believe that I was now going to inflict the same pain onto my patients, an intolerable idea.

These memories shot into my mind during my pre-operative examination of Susan. I resolved to inject long-term, local anesthetic—Marcaine—into the tonsil bed and throat muscle to induce numbness for ten to twelve hours. I learned this technique from Mr. Simon at the Whittington.

Once Susan was asleep, the area about the mouth was washed and draped by the scrub nurse. I inserted a gag to keep her mouth open and depress the tongue. Desmond helped at every step of the procedure, guiding me along. I grabbed the left tonsil with an instrument and first injected the local Lidocaine with epinephrine. The former numbed the pain, while the addition of epinephrine caused the constriction of blood vessels, minimizing bleeding. I injected the solution in a plane between the lymph tissue and the muscle of the throat, causing the plane to swell, making it easier to peel the tonsil out of its bed. Using the knife, I slowly carved out the tonsil—it was a barbaric procedure, unlike the gracefulness of performing an appendectomy. As I gained confidence working in Susan's throat, I sped up my cutting. Bleeding points were electrocoagulated to stop the oozing of blood after I took out the tonsil. I repeated the procedure on the right tonsil. After that, I injected the long-acting Marcaine. Seeing that there was no further bleeding, I removed the retractor. I ordered Demerol injections for forty-eight hours to help with pain management, in addition to the usual aspirin.

My last patient, Samantha, was a seven-year-old girl with very large adenoids at the base of the nose, obstructing the airway and leading her to snore. The adenoids, too, are lymph nodes and can get infected frequently. When enlarged, they block the eustachian tube connecting the middle ear to the back of the throat, causing middle ear infections in children. Desmond showed me how to remove them.

In total, with Desmond's help, I operated every Saturday and racked up a total of forty-two operations—mostly tonsillectomies, adenoidectomies and a variety of other small head and neck procedures such as polyps of the nose—during my six months at the Royal Ear Hospital.

18

GUILTY PLEASURES

When it comes to trust, a core dilemma of Complex-PTSD is that your longing for a relationship is in direct opposition to memories that tell you relationships aren't safe.
—Arielle Schwartz

In surgery there was no such thing as a minor case—a "minor operation." To the surgeon it was, perhaps, a minor procedure, but to the patient it was a major deal. *An operation was an operation.* Each procedure demanded the patient's trust of his surgeon, who was under the obligation to make sure everything was safe, or as the Americans said during the Gemini and Apollo space programs—all systems were "go." There was no room for errors—at least not in my book. I had to trust everyone on the team to do their part.

By early afternoon I was euphoric with the operations I had completed. Surgery was addictive. I had become a surgeon. Operating on Peter's neck, the first operation where I held the scalpel, was exhilarating. Here at the Royal Ear Hospital, I had mastered how to efficiently run a surgical ward and had established myself as a surgeon, yielding a knife to treat patients. I was full of self-assurance, high with pride, or was its hubris?

By evening, when all the doctors had gone home, I was left in charge. At times there was little to do. The patients were preoccupied with visitors, others settling in for the night, the nurses passing out meds—the ward was quiet. Like the darkness outside, the dreaded demon of loneliness, apprehension and anxiety of facing sudden emptiness gradually crept into my consciousness, retching out the core of my inner being—mental torture that replaced the high of surgery I had earlier in the day. My thoughts drifted toward wanting Hanna, craving reassurance—the balm of consolement. Was it Hanna, or just her memory? Or were these the apprehensive feelings formed in the distant past when I was unable to deal and face the "loneliness" me. I toyed with the idea of phoning Hanna, hoping she would say no—just like an addict playing with an unlit cigarette.

The craving arose from deep-seated insecurity born out of my childhood, when the inability to get Mother's love led me to another woman for comfort—at four it was my Oma. Now, the other woman was Hanna. I was conscious that the relationship with her was dangerous and futile, yet it ceaselessly drew me in like Homer's Sirens, but unlike him, I chose no wax. At Bethnal Green it was an adventure, but now, holding a scalpel, operating and staunching the flow of blood, the adventure morphed gradually toward a God-like feeling of entitlement—I *chose* not to look for wax.

Perhaps she also felt alone and disconnected from family or lacked the caring and wanting I needed so badly—I could comfort her. Should I call her? Just the thought made me despise myself.

I mustn't.

I can't.

I won't.

But I did.

I was surprised that she was willing to see me. I resigned myself to whatever power was driving my need.

We met at the top of the Casualty ramp. To be less conspicuous, she wore her nurse's uniform, her cape and her cap. We walked past waiting patients, flashing lights, rushing staff, and through the tunnels leading to the doctors' residence and crept up the back stairs, past the old bulldog guarding the entrance.

Once in my on-call room we spontaneously hugged.

"What a lovely surprise," she whispered in my ear.

"God, I've missed you."

There wasn't much more to say. It was much more than secret and forbidden sex. The craving, the urge, the lusting and loving seemed natural while a fuck was just that—a fuck. I whispered aloud, "Cunt! Eh, that's the beauty o' thee, lass!" Clinging to my shirt, head thrown back, she laughed, a throaty laugh for we had once read the naughty parts of Lawrence to each other. And, despite saying this in a measured tone, it exposed my risqué carnal self. To myself I was a stranger for I didn't and couldn't hear the warnings or see the lines I crossed—the lines of guilty pleasures.

Where I was circumspect about expressing my desires, she had no such hesitations. Her unabashed approach made me admire her and wonder where her lack of inhibition came from. She'd spice our lovemaking with whispers of "Mother Mary" when I did something that pleased her. Her response to my advances came spontaneously even when want came to call in the early morning hours, in the middle of the night, at break of dawn or just the instant before we *had* to part.

By now, I had seen many naked bodies, but Hanna's wonder was the natural way she flaunted it. When it came to nudity, she demonstrated traits opposite to mine. I had hang-ups, she displayed her body, encouraging my admiration, nay, love of it and how it provoked my response. With her, I could love without fear of embarrassment or reprimand.

She never said the words, "I love you," not even at the pulsating pinnacle of satisfaction. She held that back, for those three words implied vulnerability. I hesitated to say it although it nearly slipped through my lips during intense moments of intimacy. In Hanna's case, it was a pregnant phrase which heralded hope for a future she knew I could not give. My interest in Hanna would not change my love and commitment to Victoria.

There was a curious association between appreciating the beauty of a body, the drama of operating, and the love for a woman's body. It left me with the sense that the toxic cocktail of surgery, power, morality and hubris led some surgeons to feel they had permission to have girlfriends in addition to wives.

I soon learned via Desmond which operating theater nurse was the muse of which surgeon. It seemed a natural evolution of working together in close proximity—dealing with the daily stress: operating, healing and striving to beat back death. I began to notice the looks, the endearing comments that slipped out between particular surgeons and certain nurses, and became aware of other examples that existed among the medical community and appeared to be common knowledge.

My dream of operating on the abdomen remained elusive, but Dr. Gilliland was right, I found head and neck operations of interest. However, the breast was another surgical domain that I would become acquainted with while working at the Royal Ear Hospital.

A youngish surgeon on his team had the skill to remove the

pituitary in women with advanced or disseminated breast cancer, classified as Stage III–IV breast disease that usually occurred a few years after surgical removal of the breast cancer. Most had done well after the mastectomy but in a small fraction dormant cancer cells had subsequently metastasized throughout the body. By removing the pituitary, the pea-sized gland located in a bony hollow behind the bridge of the nose inside the skull, it was thought that the lack of those hormones would slow down the growth of hormone sensitive cancer cells and induce the metastases to shrink and die—extending the patient's life.

I usually admitted such women by 2 p.m. and compiled all the blood and X-ray tests in their charts, with greater awareness of the emotional side of apprehensive patients. I provided moral support to them, learning by listening to their medical story and avidly reading about breast cancer, regretting that I had never operated on the breast, yet yearning to one day.

The patients were moved from the ward into the operating theater at dawn, and I didn't see them again until six or seven hours later when they were awake and being rolled into their room. Following surgery, all the surgeons disappeared. Together with a group of nurses, I was left to care for the patients. Since the pituitary also produced a hormone that controlled the reabsorption of water by the kidneys, there would be a flood under each bed as the patient peed more than twenty liters of urine.

The nurse inserted a urinary catheter attached to a graduated urine-collecting bag, the floor was mopped, and I gave huge volumes of intravenous fluids to match what was lost via the kidneys. I gave injections of steroid hormones to support their blood pressure and their blood glucose, and I cared for their facial wounds—I was up most of the night stabilizing the patient. In retrospect, such unstable patients in need of intense post-operative care would have been best treated in an ICU setting—none existed at the time.

A few days after the patient was physiologically stable, she was transferred to her oncologist's care. I never found out what happened to them, whether their disease regressed as expected or how long they ultimately lived.

Only a handful of these procedures were done because the post-operative complication of providing fluids and hormones on an ongoing basis was a huge management problem. Nevertheless, addressing the whole issue of breast disease germinated in my brain.

19

DESMOND—MY BIG BROTHER

It takes two men to make one brother.
—Anonymous

Desmond was my registrar and gradually became my friend. Neither of us had brothers but found much consolation in our common backgrounds as foreign aliens in England. During our late evening meals at the Agra, we chatted about the most current news topics, but the evening invariably ended on the matter of cricket. He was a passionate follower of the world of cricket and all its intrigues, and I knew little about it.

He also enlightened me about the next steps toward becoming a surgeon. After I'd completed my job at the Royal Ear Hospital, he said I would receive a letter from the General Medical Council informing me that I was now registered as a medical practitioner in the United Kingdom. He laughed, adding, "That's such a great fucking feeling."

At the time, the route to becoming a surgeon after medical school and house officers' jobs involved passing the primary fellowship examination of London's Royal College of Surgeons. "It's a tough exam, with a pass rate of only twenty percent," he said, sipping his after-dinner masala chai. I gulped. My pulse started to race. Holy shit! *Twenty percent?* Was I going to face failure again? Had I not overcome that past demon?

"How do I prepare for the exam?"

"Reread all the stuff you learned for second MB and more," he chuckled, "and don't forget to apply. I made that mistake." He went on to explain that the exam tested the candidate's in-depth knowledge of surgical anatomy, physiology, pathology and their integration as it applied to the human body under stress of surgery or trauma.

After passing, I would embark on a three- to five-year period as a surgical registrar at various levels of seniority in general surgery. Having gained sufficient operating experience, I'd apply to sit for the final practical surgical exam. Only then would I become a Fellow of the Royal College of Surgeons.

"Imagine the acronym FRCS behind your name. That's what kept me going," Desmond said. "Passing this exam was considered easier than the primary. By then, you would be in your mid-thirties or early forties, working as a surgeon at a senior-level job, climbing the surgical career ladder to the giddy heights of a consultancy or waiting in line for "dead man's shoes" for the academic title of professor."

He scoffed, "Imagine you're still groveling to an old boss, doing all his work, getting meager pay, while your kids are on the high school cricket team!"

Desmond's guidance was greatly valued, although I didn't muddy the water by mentioning the situation with Dr. Moore and Boston, primarily because there were no equivalent arrangements for Victoria so far.

"The primary is the toughie. It's no shame if you fail. I passed on the second try, and I know someone who sat for it six times," Desmond said.

"Really? I'd be a wreck. Is there no curriculum that I need to cover to ensure I've read and learned all I need to pass?"

"No. But if you want to improve your odds, take the preparatory courses offered by the college. Mind you, they're pricy."

"I'll try to study on my own first," I retorted.

To expand my knowledge of head and neck anatomy, I began to assist Desmond in the excision of cancers of the tongue and lip. This cancer occurred most often in chronic smokers. After cutting out the cancer, a neck dissection is performed. The surgeon makes a flap of skin in the neck that is peeled back on itself to reveal the three-dimensional neck structures. The lymph glands that drain the cancer site are dissected out and removed. The anatomy is beautiful and looks like a Michelangelo diagram. Most of the preparatory dissection would be done by Desmond before Mr. Kingdom appeared. He would do the major part of the operation—removing the cancer of the voice box or the base of the tongue and the surrounding tissues. When he removed tumors of the parotid salivary gland, he made sure that the delicate branch of the facial nerve that was sandwiched between the two lobes and that controls facial expression was preserved so that the patient didn't have a droop on one side.

As I watched Mr. Kingdom work between the tightly packed vital structures in the neck, I was reminded of the mnemonics we learned to help memorize the complex anatomical relationships of the critical nerves, blood vessels and small muscles that controlled the function of the tongue, swallowing, facial expression and the voice box.

One reminder was the following: "The lingual nerve took a swerve around the hyoglossus. Well, I'll be fucked said Warton's duct, the bastard double-crossed us." The hypoglossal muscle moves the tongue, while Warton's duct is a salivary duct that drains saliva from a gland in the neck into the mouth. This ditty reminded the surgeon that the salivary duct passed twice over the hyoglossus muscle, and carelessly cutting the duct would cause saliva to drain out of the wound.

Mr. Kingdom's repertoire of head and neck operations was extensive. These procedures were long and complex cases and were relatively bloodless compared with operations of the belly. I enjoyed assisting because the anatomy of the head and neck was exquisitely beautiful. Unlike abdominal operations, it was shitless surgery. The downside was that patients with advanced head and neck surgery would receive radiation and often returned for follow-up with salivary leaks in their incisions.

"This is the 'shit' of head and neck cancer surgery," Desmond chuckled.

Saturday mornings Desmond assisted me in operating on the cases he had selected from the operative waiting list. It was a strange sensation to pick up a knife and willfully cut into a patient—deliberately be aggressive—to cure. I overcame the strongly embedded nagging from my parents telling me not to hit my elder sister at play, especially when she was a pest and when I had reached a frustration level that I could not contain. Injuring others was not allowed, but somehow, I now had permission to cut. I never quite felt secure about the patient's postoperative outcome but developed a blind faith in Desmond's reassurance that the patient would do fine during the immediate post-surgical period. At a time when I was freely wielding my scalpel and spreading my surgical wings, asserting and extending my horizon into the unknown with the fear and horror that I might harm a patient, I found Victoria's presence, her merely breathing the same air—reassuring.

As a last year medical student, Victoria was usually home on Sundays. On the weekend when I was off, we would sleep late, kiss and cuddle, have breakfast at leisure, and be together as we had been in the good old days when we had time for each other, when we *made* time for each other. When it was sunny, we walked through Regent's Park Rose Garden. Occasionally, we snuck off to the Isle of Serenity. Victoria was my security in a world full of insecurities and she banished all the thoughts of pain—the pain of abandonment that constantly rumbled beneath the surface.

When the senior registrar, Mr. Knight, a bachelor from New Zealand who I barely saw during the week, suggested he and I do "teaching rounds" together every Sunday morning from 9 a.m. until 12 p.m., I cringed. The thought of giving up my free morning when I could catch up on lost slumber and spend time with Victoria didn't make me happy. I didn't have the nerve to tell him that although I loved operating, head and neck surgery was not in my future.

"I'm afraid I go to church on Sunday mornings," was my spontaneous reply. That was well and good until he asked me which church I attended and questioned me about the sermons when we met on Monday mornings. He was suspicious. I prepared myself Sunday evenings by reading from a religious text until he stopped interrogating me.

I would look back on this rotation at the Royal Ear Hospital with satisfaction. Apart from having my own cases on Saturdays, I developed an admiration of head and neck anatomy for its absolute beauty—anatomy which I hadn't appreciated while dissecting our cadaver's neck. But I also developed an affinity for breast disease, which was almost as compelling as my desire to operate on the abdomen. And, I had gained a soul friend —Desmond.

PART IV

LONDON

SUMMER TO WINTER 1969

Like a crack in glass, it cannot be mended.
Egyptian Proverb

20

FRIENDS IN NEED

The purpose of human life is to serve and
to show compassion and the will to help others.
—Albert Schweitzer

My English School Cairo flame, Magdalena, had been traveling in Southeast Asia, accompanying an older businessman. Heading back to Brussels to resume her studies, she found herself pregnant. She called me. "If I come via London, can you help me?" I didn't like imagining her with another man. Despite the pain this caused me, I heard myself say, "Sure."

I called Desmond and as we were winding down our conversation after another scrumptious curry, I hesitantly unspooled Magdalena's plight. I explained my long-standing friendship with her while he sat across from me, sensing my discomfort. His eyes revealed a smile; he knew where the story was going. As he realized that I was trying to help a friend out of loyalty and was not the protagonist nor paternally involved, he simply said, "I'll give you a telephone number in Harley Street tomorrow."

"And how does she pay?"

He waved his hand dismissively. "They'll slip her onto the list."

I paid for our meal grateful that I had a solution for Magdalena.

The next day while doing rounds with the entire team he slipped me a piece of paper that I unfurled in the privacy of my on-call room. Next to the number, he had scribbled: "Ask for Elizabeth and tell her I gave you the number. She'll take it from there. Good luck."

A few days later, on an unusually bright and sunny late afternoon, Magdalena appeared. Victoria had not yet come home. Magdalena embraced me hesitantly, conscious of sharing a betrayal, and uncertain how I'd receive her. Neither the years nor the physical distance between us had deadened or diminished our mutual admiration, our feelings of love, our mutual ardor. And in the fundamental language that humans understand, the inseparable expressions of the human soul—our spirituality and sexuality, the common vernacular of the need to love, to be accepted and to receive love as a human and the want to be touched at our mortal core and receive assurances in return—she clung to me for forgiveness as we made love on the carpet with the sun streaming through the window onto our bare bodies.

I loved her for old times' sake.

I fucked her in my fury and rage of jealousy.

She received and loved me in her remorse.

"*Dziękuję Ci*—Thank you," is all she said as I handed her the information she needed and we took our goodbyes.

"Is anyone going with you?"

She shook her head. "God no!"

Then, she stopped to look up at me from the landing as she was climbing down the stairs and said, "*Jestem pewien, ze rozumiesz.*" I'm sure you understand.

Yes, I did. We had both grown up nurtured by people who were not our parents, leaving doubts if we were loved and leaving gigantic caverns in our souls yearning for love, acceptance and recognition. These emotions that had bound us so tightly in our youth were now being tested as we ventured along our separate paths into adulthood. Four days later, a postcard from Brussels arrived. She wrote two simple words: Thank you.

Toward the end of my six-month rotation, Mr. Kingdom asked if I'd like to help him doing a laryngectomy, removal of the voice box for cancer, on Saturday in the private wing. The venue immediately told me that this was a patient from his Harley Street practice, not one using the National Health Service. I felt complimented. In his eyes, I had made the surgical grade.

We met in the operating theater of the private wing the following morning. The anesthetist sat at the head of the operating table and had already put the patient under while he read the *Times.* To my surprise, I was Mr. Kingdom's only assistant. Typical of Mr. Kingdom's expertise, he operated swiftly, the nurse passing him the appropriate instruments while I assisted in retracting skin flaps and the three extrinsic muscles that support and positioned the larynx in the neck, hence ensuring a clear visual field. We worked in silence, in an intense and focused surgical *pas de deux* around the patient's neck. I liked operating in silence, for it helped me concentrate. By late morning, after we had removed the larynx, he excused himself and stepped out of the theater, to go and pee I presumed. On his return, he seemed agitated and preoccupied and had lost his focus and concentration.

He started to close the skin. I watched him for a couple of stitches. "Aren't you going to close the three underlying muscle layers?" I asked. He looked up, stared into my eyes, and I saw the momentary terror of the realization of his error.

"Good God. He'd have blown his neck wide open and died on taking his first breath." He cut out the skin sutures and started to close the underlying muscle layers. His focus had returned. I continued to assist.

Feeling glad I had the confidence to speak out about my surgical concern and happy that my helpful question was well received, I was surprised when in the changing room, the boss slipped me a £5 note. I wavered. Seeing his face at my vacillation, I realized this was not fee splitting but a gesture of gratitude. By speaking up, I had saved his patient's life, spared him an investigation, and, perhaps, the demise of his life's practice.

I had learned at Mass General that every member of the surgical team, no matter their status, was responsible for the patient's welfare. If a procedure doesn't look right, I learned to speak up, regardless of the humiliation and shame that may come from being wrong.

Walking home, I recognized that challenging authority, in this case my surgical superior, hadn't been easy, but I had done it. My self-worth had been beaten up during my early years by Opa, the autocrat, my father, the perfectionist, and, more recently, Rosenheim, the rotter. When it came to surgery, by speaking up to Mr. Kingdom, I had at that moment overcome my shaky self-esteem and fear of possible embarrassment.

On this rotation, I had gained the buoyancy to pick up the knife myself and cut another human, not to harm but to heal. As a budding surgeon, my words and actions mattered. Kudos boosted my self-confidence and bolstered my dignity. I saw my mentors, Professor Pilcher and Mr. Kingdom, as Imhotep, the ancient Egyptian god of medicine, and Dr. Gilliland as

Hippocrates, the Greek physician. They lighted my determination to become a healer and surgeon.

I floated home along Euston Street. Trailing me was a stranger I'd eventually acknowledge as the hubris of a surgeon.

21

A REQUEST

I do not care so much what I am to others as I care what I am to myself.

—Michel de Montaigne

As Desmond mentioned, the letter from the General Medical Council arrived. I was now registered as a medical practitioner in the United Kingdom, and it felt good. As a registered medical practitioner, I could place the acronym MBBS (Bachelor of Medicine, Bachelor of Surgery), in addition to LMSSA (the diploma Licentiate in Medicine and Surgery of the Society of Apothecaries), after my name on my stationery. I chose only the former. Despite my father boasting two PhDs, he could not match me in the medical field, and I planned to outstrip him in recognition. I was aiming to become a surgeon and to have the acronym FRCS—Fellow of the Royal College of Surgeons—or if I got the chance to train in America, FACS, Fellow of the American College of Surgeons.

With the MBBS, or simply put, MB, I belonged to a venerable profession. An overwhelming feeling of success swept over me; six years after leaving Manchester as an immature youth, I had attained my label of "doctor" in the late spring of 1969, a few months after my twenty-fourth birthday. I was ready to face the medical challenges and vagaries of human ailments.

Victoria, too, had now passed her finals, concluding five years of medical school. Without taking a breath, she was immediately thrust into fulfilling her one-year obligatory house jobs or internships before she too would get a letter from the council. We would both be licensed practitioners. In the meantime, for the next year, she would be cooped up: six months at Westminster doing a pediatric house job and then six months as a Casualty officer at Queen Mary's Hospital, Roehampton. These were all geographically removed from Albany Street. She would be living every other night and every other weekend in the hospital, apart from two weeks' holiday; if our schedules didn't synchronize most of the time, we would be like two individuals trying to live together, each in our own spheres. Love would help us survive this demanding period of chronic separation.

Despite these vital transitions of triumph in our lives, we didn't celebrate. We didn't take the moment to savor our achievements, to renew our commitment to each other since we were now at a higher personal and professional plane. There was no time, or more precisely, we didn't make the time. How could we?

We should have found a way to salute each other's growth and reaffirm our plans and goals for our lives together. We should have gone on a much-needed holiday together somewhere in the sun, where we could lie on a beach and savor each other, rekindle our passion and recapture the feelings that we once had for each other. Instead, we continued our uphill path toward some long-term professional goals that, from time to time, included the dream of America. We were both overwhelmed with our imminent tasks—she her house jobs and I the primary fellowship exam.

Studying alone most of the day was a mind killer. All the anxieties I had lived with, cooped up in my room at Commonwealth Hall while studying for my basic science exam, resurfaced. I welcomed distractions, thinking that the primary was several months away. As I wandered, aimlessly studying, being bored, waiting for my beloved and quenching my loneliness by occasionally seeing Hanna, another letter arrived. This one was from my GP, Dr. B. He invited me to visit him in his solo practice office in Camden Town, some twenty minutes from our flat. We had last met when he made a house call after the UCH Casualty officer had diagnosed me with infectious mononucleosis.

Sitting on the crowded bus with the evening commuters, heading to Camden Town in North London on my way to Dr. B's practice, I was curious why he had asked to see me.

"Are you better?" was his opening remark when I entered his office.

"Yes, much."

"Wasn't it a few months ago? Yes, I remember I made a house call. You were sent home from serving as House Officer at the ear hospital because you had Mono—Infectious Mononucleosis. Yes, you were quite sick. It took you six weeks to get over it. Isn't that right? Six weeks at home."

"Yep. Six boring weeks. Mind you I don't recall much, as I slept a lot."

We were in his upstairs examining room. When he stood up to greet me, I noticed that he was younger than I had remembered—perhaps ten years older than me. He, too, was a graduate of UCH and had built up an impressive family practice with nearly two thousand registered patients. I could hear his secretary, Jenny, downstairs pottering about. Outside, it was getting dark. She popped her head around his office door. "I've locked up," she said, and waving a sheet of paper, "Here's the list of the two patients you'll need to visit when you've finished with Dr. Meguid." She closed his door. We were alone again. Rain started to drum against the windows.

He produced a bottle of sherry from underneath the sink. "Would you like a glass?" I declined. Taking a sip, he looked over the rim of the glass and said, "You were quite ill," and after a pause, he said, "the Epstein-Barr herpes virus spreads primarily by saliva—some kiss, eh?" and chuckled.

I asked, "Have you ever seen patients get lymphoma or head and neck cancer later in life from this virus, as is commonly claimed?"

"No. I wouldn't worry about it."

Apart from the rush hour traffic, the room fell into an awkward silence. I studied his face, trying to read his mood and what was on his mind. In the darkening room his face caught the yellow streetlight coming through the window, which rattled slightly with the brisk wind and each passing double decker. The glare from the streetlight dramatized his suddenly contorted face, resembling a gargoyle. He uttered in a pained voice, "I found this man lying between my wife's legs, kissing her." His voice, loaded with venom, hissed, "Disgusting."

My book knowledge had not covered this type of confession. Then, more soberly, he repeated, "Disgusting . . . kissing her . . . down there."

He emptied his sherry glass. "I need a break, six weeks, to figure things out. Will you do a locum for me? I'll pay you £36 per week."

I was taken aback. "I've arranged to do an anatomy proctorship at University College and then planned to attend the lecture series at the Royal College of Surgeons before sitting for the surgical primary fellowship exam," I replied, less an answer than explanation as I thought aloud. I wondered how such an interruption would impinge on my study plans and my progress in preparing for the primary exam. Would this also affect my limited time with Victoria? I hesitated. In the silence that followed, he lit his desk lamp.

"Well, what do you think? It's a very nice practice. You would come here from nine to twelve and three to six. Jenny copes with the patients, paperwork, and the office. She's good . . . makes things easy for me."

In the hush broken by passing buses, I tried to think what I'd exactly have to do.

He must have taken my silence as a form of reluctance and to sweeten the deal he said, "I'll arrange that you're not on weekend calls and you'd have the practice's car at your disposal. By the way, twice a week you'll cover Grosvenor House Hotel for medical emergencies between five in the evening until eight in the morning. It's good money—you get to bill the patients directly."

I agreed, more out of compassion and curiosity than the inducement of three times my usual salary. Maybe I was also procrastinating, not wanting to study for yet another exam. I started the following Monday.

22

THE GP PRACTICE

It is the surgeon's duty to tranquillize the temper, to beget cheerfulness, and to impart confidence of recovery.
—Astley Cooper

Ten minutes before Jenny unlocked the practice door, she stood next to me at Dr. B.'s desk, pointing to a stack of weathered and well-fingered index cards. "You'll see these patients this morning. Donald saw some of them last week. They're returning for follow-up."

"What am I seeing them for?"

"It's on the card. Others are coming in today with new complaints. Try to stick to ten minutes per patient if you don't want to fall too far behind, as I have a luncheon appointment. If you need me, press this button," she said, pointing to one under the desktop, "and I'll come up. If I'm busy, I'll phone you. The last half-hour is for walk-ins. When you've finished, I'll give you a list of patients for house calls." As she turned toward the office door, she added, "Don't forget to write a note on each patient's card." And with "good luck," she left me to figure out the patient records.

Dr. B.'s handwriting was neat and slanted to the right. He abbreviated many medical terms, leaving me to decipher out what he meant.

At 9 a.m., Mrs. Beatty, a fifty-three-year-old widow, coughed her way into the office. She held a small towel into which she spat.

"I can't breathe," she said. "Last week, visiting my grandchildren in Belfast, I got caught up in the Troubles and was gassed by our boys. It burns with each breath." Pointing to her chest, "And I bring up a lot of spit, doctor, all the time. Imagine. Gassed by my people," she added indignantly. She coughed again, cleared her throat, and spat phlegm into the towel. "It's really awful, doctor. You know what I mean." I got up and listened to her lungs. She had squeaking noises with each breath and coughed vigorously when she breathed deeply.

"You probably have an inflammation of your lung, some irritation from the gas." I prescribed her an antibiotic and wrote on a prescription pad: Please evaluate and treat for CS tear gas exposure. "Take this note to Casualty at UCH and hand it to the nurse. They will treat you further." She stood up, adjusted her clothes, thanked me and left. I annotated her card as follows: Chemical exposure to lung—probably CS gas. Sent to UCH. I dated and signed.

Mrs. Anson walked in, her eight-year-old daughter in tow. "I think she has lice, doctor. She constantly scratches her head."

"What's your name?"

"Jill."

Approaching, I asked, "How long have you had this?"

Looking up, her mother answered, "A week."

I parted her light-colored hair, looked on the scalp, around the hairline and the nape of the neck, seeking the white shells of nits. "Your mum's right," I said. "You have head lice, Jill."

"Well, she didn't get it from my house. I keep it spotless. You must have got it from those Irish kids you play with," said Mrs. Anton in an accusatory tone.

"You will need to wash her hair with this medicated shampoo," I wrote out a script and handed it to her. "If you have other children, they will all have to be treated too. And wash the linen."

Addressing her daughter, Mrs. Anson said, "Now, what do you say to the doctor?"

"Thank you," Jill said shyly.

I saw Mrs. Wesley next. She looked depressed and wanted a refill of her prescription.

"Why do you take 5 mg prednisone, Mrs. Wesley?"

"Don't know. The doctor gave it to me as a tonic for my moods." I thumbed through her cards, looking for her symptoms or a diagnosis warranting the prescription of a steroid. I could not find it. An image of Mrs. Sloan, my defiant patient at Bethnal Green, floated by, and I wondered if Dr. B. was prescribing this drug for a lonely woman who often came to complain of chronically vague symptoms.

"Do you really need it, Mrs. Wesley?"

"I feel good when I take it. And the doctor gave it to me." She added forcefully, "He is very good, you know."

I wrote another script, limiting the quantity of pills. Handing it to her I said, "I'll see you again in a fortnight. Make an appointment with the secretary downstairs." I noted my action on her card.

The next patient was a middle-aged smoker. Mr. Elliott was a postman. "I need a letter excusing me from work last Thursday and Friday. I wasn't well."

"What was the problem?"

He hesitated. "I just didn't feel well, doctor," he restated shifting in his chair. I looked at him skeptically and then through his scant records and could not find evidence of any chronic illness. On examining him, the only findings were limited to his chest.

"Did you come and see Dr. B.?"

"No, I was too sick."

"How long have you been smoking? And how much do you smoke each day?" I asked.

"Since I left the army. About two packs a day."

"I want you to go to UCH and get a chest X-ray. Come back in a couple of days."

"Yes, but I need a note excusing me from work," he repeated.

"Well, man, what was your problem?" I said, irritated and raising my voice. "You can't just not go to work and expect me to write you a note. I'm not your mother. I'll see you after your X-ray," I said, standing up. "Perhaps, then, I can write you a note."

"Dr. B. would have given me a note," he repeated forcefully. "You youngsters think you know it all." With that, he stormed out, slamming the door. I suspected he had been picketing in the national postal strike while I was not getting my mail for a week. I should have added: *If you do your job and deliver my mail, perhaps I'll write you a note.* I was more than irritated because the trash was also not being collected and was piling up. It seemed that most union workers throughout England were on strike.

As the morning progressed with one patient after another, I realized there was little I could do other than write prescriptions or refer patients to consultants at UCH. My frustration gradually rose. This was not my type of medicine, not my type of job.

Late in the morning, the phone rang, and Jenny informed me that one of Dr. B.'s patients was climbing up the stairs with his elderly father, who was not registered with the practice.

I pulled up a second chair for Mr. Christakos' father, who

seemed in great distress, while his son, a middle-aged businessman, fretted over him. "My father is visiting from Cyprus, and he can't pee. Can you *please* help him?" he said in a heavy Greek accent. I motioned for the father to lie down on the examining couch. His lower abdomen was distended and dull to percussion, indicating an enlarged bladder, almost up to his navel. He groaned with each gentle prodding. Suspecting that he had urinary retention, I rolled him onto his left side and performed a rectal exam, finding an enlarged, craggy prostate consistent with a cancer. I could have easily relieved him of the discomfort if I had a catheter, but there was none. My frustration increased further, for the office was not equipped for interventional therapy.

I started to write a referral addressed to DRD, the consultant urologist at UCH who had me do the many rectals when I was a student, when I noticed Mr. Christakos sliding a ten-pound note across the desk, pleading, "Please help my father." In his culture, like in Egypt, a bribe would be necessary for treatment. I held up my hand to stop him, and he pocketed the note. Jenny arranged for an ambulance to the hospital.

I had one call to make during lunch break. I disliked house calls; the idea of entering a sick stranger's home made me uncomfortable. In addition, I felt impotent at the likelihood that I could not perform a comprehensive examination, lacking ancillary medical support.

Mrs. Petersen, a widow in her late seventies, lived in the shadow of the practice. The front door was unlocked and I entered.

"Hello? This is the doctor," I yelled.

A feeble voice beckoned me to the upstairs bedroom. Her house was dark and damp, and the stairs creaked as I climbed. There was a faint odor of violet water, failing to mask the smell of stale smoke.

Mrs. Petersen sat semi-propped up in bed. She had a

constellation of symptoms, including wheezing and coughing up a lot of yellow sputum. Next to her bed was an ashtray filled with cigarette butts, which made me think of bronchitis as a likely diagnosis. I examined her. She had a low-grade fever and some swelling of her lower legs, and throughout my exam, she coughed, making it difficult to hear her lungs.

"Mrs. Petersen, you have an attack of acute bronchitis. I'm going to admit you to the chest service at UCH."

"Oh no. Who's going to take care of my cat?" she said. "Dr. B. usually treats me at home whenever I have a flare up."

"You have to stop smoking. This is very serious. I'll give you an antibiotic. Is there someone who can get this prescription to the chemist?"

She shook her head. "My son is coming to visit next weekend," she said between each breath.

"I'll phone your script to the chemist and call a social worker to see you tonight. Do you have enough food, or should she also get some bread, cheese, and tomatoes for you?"

As I left, Mrs. Petersen's tabby cat scurried up the stairs, squeezing past my legs.

During afternoon office hours, I saw patients with complaints similar to the ones I had encountered in the morning. I was increasingly uncomfortable with the many patients who came merely to get a prescription refill. Often, I could not figure out their diagnosis in Dr. B.'s records. I had no evening house calls on my first day.

At home, I tried to telephone Victoria. I wanted to hear her voice, to feel close to her, to feel her presence, to ground me after a frustrating day. I needed her. I left a message with a nurse for her to call me. Then, I sat down to face reality: I had to develop study plans in preparation for the primary.

The next day, I arrived early, primarily to get a parking space for the Morris Minor in front of the practice on High Street. Jenny was already preparing the three-by-five records of the patients I was to see.

"How did your visit to Mrs. Petersen go yesterday?"

Giving Jenny her record, I related the events.

"Yes, social service phoned earlier to establish visiting her and also to pick up her medication."

This type of practice in medicine could not sustain me. I felt useless; I was a doer, I needed to see patients I could operate on. Only then would I feel fulfilled. Surgery was my vocation. There was no way to back out of my commitment. It was going to be a long six weeks.

23

MORAL DILEMMAS

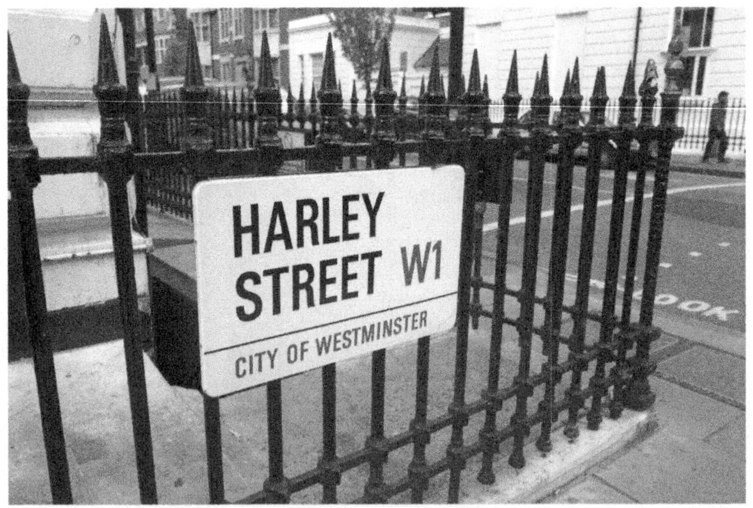

Thinglass / Shutterstock.com

Our very lives depend on the ethics of strangers,
and most of us are always strangers to other people.
—Bill Moyers

The following morning, Jenny barged into the office before my first patient and paused in front of the desk.

"Your 10:30 a.m. just called. Her flight was late. She's taking a taxi from Heathrow straight here."

"Who's the patient? And what's this airport business?"

"It's today, remember? They arrive every Tuesday usually around nine-thirty. Didn't Dr. B tell you before he left?"

"Tell me what?"

"The referrals he gets. Some practitioners in the Twin Cities in America send patients to London for an abortion. You see them . . ." She lay a printed sheet on the desk. "Sign this. She'll need it for her two o'clock appointment at the private clinic, and she is running late."

"What abortion?"

She looked inquisitively and said, "Don't they teach you anything in medical school?"

Was she being funny?

"Give me a break. I just started this job yesterday," I argued. "This sounds more like your practice issue than my medical schooling. Anyway, I'm not signing anything until I've seen the patient and I know what's it about!"

"Oh dear," she said. "Donald said you were a free-spirited youngster, but I don't think he thought you were going to change his practice." Stepping back, she lowered her voice, "Are you, doctor?"

Standing up I stepped in front the desk to face her. "Now look here, I'm his *locum*. His patients and this practice are now my responsibility," I said emphatically, "I do not intend to change anything. Neither am I going to sign a so-called abortion letter without knowing or first examining a patient. It's bad enough you give me refill scripts of meds to sign for dubious diagnoses for patients I've not seen."

"Oh dear." She viewed me over her glasses and placed a hand on her right hip. At that moment, she looked older than her forty years of age.

"It is 1969, and they've landed a man on the moon, but you can't get a legal abortion in America. Get it? Some docs in Minnesota refer them to Dr. B. He sends them to a psychiatrist. Your signed affidavit, together with his, and she gets it done. Hey presto! Tomorrow morning, you'll check her out, then she flies back. All right?"

Putting her other hand on her left hip, she added, "Now, do you get it? So, don't get your knickers twisted, just sign." As she spoke her voice became progressively louder.

Livid. I felt trapped. Raising my voice to meet her pitch, I nearly shouted, "And . . . that's . . . legal?"

"Sure," she said adamantly. "Just like if it's one of our own patients who needs it." Taking a step forward, she added in her London accent, "Now please sign, so that she won't be late for her appointment."

"I thought I knew where I stood on this issue. But the way I'm forced to be drawn into some scheme makes me very leery. How do I know she is pregnant, for one thing?"

"Really, doctor?" she said in exasperation. "Do you think some MD over there is going to send a patient over here with an imaginary pregnancy?"

I was fuming. Never had I been treated like this. I was twenty-five years old, a married man, a licensed physician, part of an honorable profession, despite this being my real first job. I expected a modicum of respect.

"This is outrageous! Think pseudocyesis," I hissed. "I'd look pretty silly referring a patient who wasn't pregnant. Now please get a pregnancy test and let me know the result."

"She *is* at least ten to twelve weeks!" She bellowed in my face as she stepped forward.

"How the hell... do... you... know?"

"They said *so* when they referred her from Minneapolis for the appointment. It's all in the paperwork you have to sign."

There was a silence as we each stood our ground. Turning to sit down I said dismissively, "I want to read it first."

"For heaven's sakes. It's standard stuff! I've run this practice for years. Dr. B just signs." Without waiting for a reply, she added, "We're behind. The waiting room is filling up."

"*I'll* buzz *you* after I've read it," I replied tersely as she turned and stormed out of the office.

The professor of obstetrics who supervised my obstetric course at UCH had preached incessantly in his Australian accent about women's rights. He had warned about the nightmare of back street abortionists and the risk of females left sterile or, worse, bleeding to death. He condemned and preached to us about the purveyors of guilt and hypocrisy, the buggerers of altar boys, the enslavers and subjugators of women, the countless unwanted children and progressive, world-wide poverty. While pursuing postgraduate studies at Yale, he was perplexed that American woman would blindly accept the male-determined fate of their bodies. As a medical student, I was indoctrinated and uncritically supportive of his more progressive views. But I had serious qualms about the choice of abortion. I had experienced the firsthand pain of discovering Mother's intent to abort me. It may be a woman's right to choose, but there was more to this issue. What about the male partner? I guess my father objected. Thanks to him, I am alive today. I wish I didn't find myself in this predicament.

I looked at the document Jenny had placed before me.

Affidavit
Sir,
I, Dr. Michael Meguid, have duly examined Debra Ann Egdahl, and I have counseled her on her condition. She is estimated to be twelve weeks pregnant. Further, I have discussed at length with her the mitigating reasons for seeking a termination. She understands that since abortion is a safe medical procedure that carries relatively few physical or psychological risks…

I skipped a paragraph.

Finally, I have emphasized to her the alternative choice of adoption, and since she seeks a termination, she agrees to family counseling and to birth control measures, until such time that she is in a position to have a family…

The letter ended with the following:

I concur with and endorsed her wish for a termination. To ensure welfare of her mental health, I am referring her for a psychiatric evaluation.

Sincerely,
Michael Meguid MB BS

I took a deep breath and signed, a vortex of mixed feelings flying around me. I buzzed Jenny. To my surprise, she ushered an unaccompanied Ms. Egdahl into my office. She was a petite Caucasian woman who sat across from me, stone-faced and silent. She wore no make-up but was more elegantly dressed than the often-dowdy late middle-aged patients in my waiting room. She handed me a document showing the result of her American positive pregnancy test and then dutifully answered all the questions raised in the affidavit. She stated that in her mind, an abortion would solve her problem—adding that without which, she would probably lose her job.

Before I could clinically examine her, Jenny walked in once more and announced, "Her taxi is waiting."

Hesitantly, I rose and wished Ms. Egdahl good luck. My watch showed that eight minutes had passed. By tomorrow, I imagined, her nightmare would be over, and her previous life would resume once more, uninterrupted.

The next morning, Wednesday, at 9 a.m., Ms. Egdahl sat across the desk, handbag on her lap. She was calm. I'd imagined someone who had her insides scraped would be in pain and have some discomfort or even be distraught from what I perceived must be an immense emotional trauma. If she was, it did not show.

I proceeded with some general health questions. My voice faltered for a second at the futility of the exercise. She sat up, "How much do I owe you?" This threw me off. Presumably, Dr. B had a long-standing arrangement with his connections in Minnesota, which, of course, he had not divulged. I was curious what Ms. Egdahl had paid in Harley Street but didn't ask. I, as a GP, was now part of the British National Health Service, free universal health care. My thoughts drifted briefly to Magdalena. She, too, had been beneficiary of health care's charity.

"Nothing," I heard myself say. "You owe me nothing. Buy yourself a nice dress before you fly back."

Tears filled her eyes. Her stoic façade cracked for a brief

moment. Feebly, I offered her a box of tissues, feeling acutely embarrassed—there was much more to this issue than I had realized. Within moments, she composed herself, rose, thanked me and left.

My next patient, Mr. Partridge, had a surgical belly, with cramps and bleeding stools, complications from long-standing ulcerative colitis, dutifully enunciated by his wife, who accompanied him. Based on my examination, I suspected he probably had an abscess in his abdomen that needed draining. I dashed off a brief note addressed to the Casualty physician at UCH with a sense of pride at having made a worthy diagnosis, one that required proper surgical intervention. I wished I could do the procedure myself.

By the end of my first week, I became a connoisseur of mainly trivial and medico-social complaints, dispensing pills and sick notes, treating coughs, colds, and psychosomatic ailments. Anything vaguely surgical and of interest to me was referred to the hospital. On top of that, I was uncomfortable at some of the seemingly unsavory practices that I was drawn into and which I could not control—refilling prescriptions for undefined diagnoses and dispensing abortions. Was I unscrupulous or just naïve about the real issues that physicians faced in a family practice? Was I in a position to judge Dr. B.'s behavior? I lived in a glass house, too, a different type but glass all the same. *Judge not, that ye be not judged*, came to mind, and I certainly was no angel. Had I not sexually *transgressed* on several occasions, had I not *lied* to get out of a pharmacology experiment and *lied* to get a second key for 65 Gower Street for Victoria? And had I not *helped myself* to a cup of tea from the doctor's lounge to which I was not entitled? On the other hand, had I not *confessed* to Dr. James about not knowing neuroanatomy, and *confessed* to knowing a patient in the crucial surgical examination, which cost me the Lister prize.

In the different cultures I had inhabited, moral values were not necessarily similar. I had navigated the ethical relativism of the Egyptian gray-zone life, post-war German hidden truths, and, now, the verities of British medical morality. Where exactly was the truth on any matter? What were the principles, and who dictated them? Where had I read the quote, "And the truth shall set you free," and who had said it? I wish it were true. Nevertheless, by the end of the first week I felt a sense of empowerment. I was a real doctor and despite the vagaries of the medical conditions I had seen, I felt I was able to help people. It was an impressive and exalted feeling.

On Saturday morning during breakfast, a blue envelope fell through our front door mail drop. It looked professional, with my address typed but without a return address. Ten crisp £5 notes cascaded onto the floor when I opened it.

Victoria gathered them and said, "Look at this."

I stared at her with a growing sense of mixed emotions that included avarice and discomfort. What line was I now being dragged across? What line was transgressed? Had I become an unwitting pawn or a corrupt mercenary? Still, being poor students, we welcomed the money, yet would I have returned it if I knew who had sent it? I felt trapped and mentioned the probable source of the funds to Victoria. We suggested that we not bank it but instead return it to the practice.

On Monday morning, I asked Jenny, "Are the funds mine or that of the practice?" Agitated, she looked away and fiddled with the papers and pens on her desk. She seemed alarmed that I had raised the issue of money. "No. You signed the affidavit. So, you keep what you get," she replied tersely.

As we talked, a Mrs. Beth S. Norseman was boarding a transatlantic flight bound for London from St. Paul. She told her husband she and her girlfriend were going to London on a week's shopping trip. The 707 would leave its white contrails, its vapor trail across the blue Atlantic sky, delivering her to the practice by 9 a.m. tomorrow morning to collect her affidavit dutifully signed by me and attesting that she was pregnant. A few days later, while Mrs. Norseman and her girlfriend were breaking their fast at the Connaught Hotel before going shopping at Harrods, another blue envelope fell through my mail drop. If abortions were legal, as Jenny claimed, why was there an inducement?

That Friday morning, I saw Beatrice, an eighteen-year-old shop assistant in the High Street haberdashery near the practice who entered my office and stood some distance in front of my desk.

"I'm pregnant," she declared, firmly, adding, "About twelve weeks."

"I see. Come and sit down."

"No. You, like all the others, will try and talk me out of it." She remained standing.

I looked up at her. "How many periods have you missed?"

"They were always irregular—a couple I imagine."

"Have you noticed more tenderness of your breasts, nausea, or mood swings—"

"I was tested. I'm pregnant."

"Were the results confirmed?"

"Look, my boyfriend and I decided on an abortion. We don't want an unplanned baby, only when we marry," she said, adding, "Soon."

"Beatrice, as your doctor, I'm just trying to make sure you'll be all right. I have no personal opinion in this matter. Since I have to sign the papers for you, there are some things I need to cover, such as adoption, birth control and so on."

"Collin and I have discussed all these things, and we don't want anything or anyone, neither your secretary nor you, to stop us."

"And marriage?"

"It's none of your business. Anyway, Collin will be filing for a divorce."

Jenny had told me that Beatrice was coming and that she and Collin, her boyfriend, had their minds set on a termination. "I tried to persuade her otherwise," Jenny added, "But they are adamant, so don't confuse her." Collin came with her but waited downstairs while Beatrice climbed the stairs to my office. I sensed that she thought that I was encroaching into her personal life. I backed off.

I was unable to develop a rapport with Beatrice while she stood in front of me, refusing the proffered chair. Failing to make a medical connection despite my empathy, I signed the affidavit. She took it and withdrew, saying in a triumphant voice, "I have an appointment at the Marie Stopes Clinic."

Here was a prime example of what the professor of obstetrics had preached while I was at UCH. In the era of enlightened women, the ethos was that they had the right to control their body and decide the fate of their pregnancy, free of paternalistic medical interference. His last words in the tutorial rang through my ears: "By the time a woman has made the painful decision to have an abortion, in my experience, she has gone through hell." Beatrice was my patient but didn't need a seemingly omnipotent doctor to tell her what to do. She was determined to terminate the growth in her uterus.

No blue envelope appeared during the next ten days. In a twisted way, I wondered, "Jenny? Do you know if Beatrice had her procedure?"

"Oh yes. She was tearful but otherwise seemed quite happy when I spoke to her."

"Did she call in?"

"No. I called her. She had been seen by the obstetrician in the clinic and did not want a follow-up appointment here."

During the following weeks, I settled into Dr. B's medical practice and managed to develop a limited study routine, facing my surgical texts and stoked by the concern of the approaching primary exam. I was not investing as much time into my preparations as I should. Perhaps I was doing this willingly, fearing failure of the exam—one I *would* fail and suffer, facing and wrestling with my internal demons if I did not apply myself.

A few weeks later, Beatrice and Collin barged into my office. She was in a rage. Her hair was unkempt and tears streamed down her face. Collin held her back as she attempted to rush at me.

She yelled, "You made me have the abortion. Thanks to you, I lost my child."

I shoved my chair backward, trying to escape her lunging.

Collin continued to restrain her, saying, "It's not his fault, dear. Not his fault." She continued to threaten me, plunging forward to attack me.

"You murderer, you evil pig." She picked up the paperweight on my desk and threw it. I saw the deep hurt in her eyes as I ducked.

Her distressed screams resonated throughout the practice, bringing Jenny up the stairs. She escorted an anguished, weeping Beatrice out of my office. My heart rate slowly sank back to normal as I straightened my clothes.

"I have to talk to you, doctor," Collin said, brushing his hair back. "She's upset. I did not go with her. She didn't want me to. She now accuses me of not being there when she needed me. At first, she was fine. We both felt relieved. Then it started . . . the weeps and lots of tears. She is like that . . . doctor." He looked away.

"Do sit down, man," I said, exasperated.

He took the chair. "I wasn't ready to be a father to her baby. I'm married and have young ones of my own. My wife would throw me out and I wouldn't see my youngsters. If her parents found out, they might prevent Bea from seeing me. She wanted the baby." He hesitated. "We chose the easy way out." Stuttering and choking up he said, "I thought we knew what we were doing."

"Why did she want the baby? Did she think it would force you to leave your wife?"

"I don't know, really, doctor," Collin said looking at my desk. "It's my fault. It was mainly my decision . . . I pressured her . . . she's Catholic." Then he admitted, "Her pregnancy was the problem and abortion the only solution we could think of—at least that I could think of."

After another brief pause, I got up. "We'll arrange for both of you to see someone." And with that, he too stood up and quietly left.

The summary reports I received from the psychiatric social worker stated that Beatrice remained distressed. She stopped working. I was asked to prescribe an anti-depressant. Their relationship deteriorated as regret, denunciation and guilt consumed them. Blaming him, she stopped seeing Collin.

I met Collin a couple of times while shopping in the high street. He felt angry, helpless and riddled with remorse. Raised a Methodist, he told me that he had become more involved in his church "To help me forget and seek forgiveness." He made no mention of his wife, and since she wasn't my patient, I could not ask about her or the state of their relationship.

The Beatrice crisis played out throughout the last few weeks of my locum while I focused on my surgical studies in preparation for the examination. I felt bad for Beatrice because I had so glibly followed medical dictum as I had been taught when I should have spent more time with Beatrice and focused more closely on her motivations for getting pregnant and for demanding an abortion. My signing an affidavit for termination reinforced the law that a woman had the right to self-determine about what happened to her body. She was an individual whom I had to respect, not a diagnosis.

Collin, her partner, was the other half of the story. He, too, should have been interrogated to see his motives and future plans to prevent similar pregnancies and his degree of support for his partner. The problem was that he wasn't my patient. The lessons of the emotional fall-out and its lasting effect on each partner depended on their psychological resilience. The affidavit asked about counseling. Should a similar situation arise, I would require counseling to begin before signing. This consideration was not to negate the abortion but to fully inform the patient or the couple what might follow—relief, grief, regret, anxiety and a permanent scarring of the soul.

I wondered if I was too emotionally involved—more than a physician might or should be. In sorting out my thoughts, I was once again grateful I had not been aborted. I was sad for the young American women who had to come here to rectify their problem. They were the lucky, affluent ones. Women crossing the Atlantic were brave, as brave and resilient as the very young Irish girls who crossed the Mersey and took a train down to London to write the script of their destiny. It was a sad state of affairs that women in America had to come here because they didn't have a choice at home. I would support them.

24

UPROOTING A TURNIP

AUGUST 1969

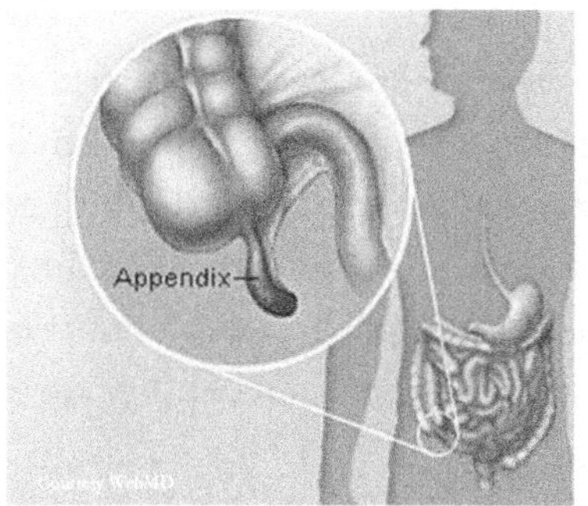

If the operation is difficult, you aren't doing it right.
—Anonymous

On an early evening during my GP locum, the family in Suite 2432 at the Grosvenor House Hotel telephoned for a doctor. The symptoms related to me by Mr. Erdman sounded ominous. His fifteen-year-old son, Timothy's, stomachache had worsened over the last four hours. Would I come as soon as possible?

When I arrived, Timothy lay on the bedspread, his parents

hovering anxiously about. Timothy's eyes apprehensively tracked my approach as his father ushered me into the suite. The family had driven down from Yorkshire, starting shortly after an early breakfast. They had planned a night at a West End theater—front row seats for *Hair*—followed by dinner at the Savoy.

"We thought we'd show him some of the finer sides of life now that he's becoming a man," Mrs. Erdman said. "Tomorrow, both my men are heading to Savile Row." Mr. Reedman stood by her, wordless, weighing me up. Had he expected an elderly physician?

"Timmy didn't eat his lunch but drank a little Glucose-Aid, felt nauseated, then lay in the backseat of the Bentley," she prattled on nervously as Mr. Erdman led me to the bathroom, where I washed my hands.

My shoes sank into the deep pile carpet, a level of luxury I had not seen in any of the hotels within my budget. Timmy's eyes were sunken, his face clammy. He told me that he'd eaten breakfast—fried eggs, fried tomato, fried black pudding, and fried bread—just to please his mum, even though it was tasteless and he hadn't had his usual morning bowel movement.

"My pain started in the pit of my stomach," he said pointing to the area about his belly button. He thought his nausea was due to carsickness because of his dad's new Bentley, but he'd never suffered from it before. When his father had made a pit stop in Cambridge, he had not felt like getting out of the car to visit his uncle's college. Neither the chapel, nor the stained-glass windows, nor the manicured gardens held any charm for him. "I refused lunch, feeling certain I'd vomit."

Timothy's temperature was one hundred degrees Fahrenheit. After I examined his throat to exclude tonsillitis, I listened to his lungs and heart. He said weakly, "The pain is here now," pointing to the lower right side of his belly.

I gently started to examine Timothy's abdomen with my

warmed hand, constantly talking to him about school, his hobbies, and friends as I had done when examining patients in Casualty to distract him while intently watching his face for signs of pain induced by my examination.

Throughout, Mr. Erdman and his wife watched apprehensively from the foot of the bed, occasionally exchanging a quiet word or two.

I palpated the right lower quadrant progressively deeper and saw the pain reflected in Timothy's face. I suddenly released the pressure and Timothy groaned, "Ouch."

I said I was sorry and meant it; I did not add that I knew exactly how he felt, for I had the same illness when I was eleven.

Turning to his parents, I said, "I suspect that your son has appendicitis. He will need an emergency operation. I recommend Mr. Rodney Maingot, the most eminent consultant abdominal surgeon in London."

Sensing that Mr. and Mrs. Erdman seemed apprehensive of my youth, I suggested they confer with their GP back home about my referral. When they left to make the call, I performed a rectal exam on Timmy; his intra-abdominal right lower quadrant was tender, and my probing elicited pain that was distinct from the discomfort of the exam, confirming my diagnosis. Mr. Erdman returned with the GP's blessing. By now, it was 6:30 p.m., the height of private surgical consultation hours.

I phoned Mr. Maingot in Harley Street, maneuvering past his protective office manager. Eventually, I was put through to the famous man himself. After briefly introducing myself, I related Timothy's history and the physical findings. Mr. Maingot agreed that the most likely diagnosis was appendicitis. His secretary would arrange for Timothy's admission to St. George's Hospital, which was nearby at Hyde Park Corner. She would also schedule his case with the operating theater, and

Mr. Maingot would meet the patient and his parents around 8 p.m. In the meantime, he would order blood tests.

When I received the call in my office, I had never actually performed an appendectomy.

"Would you like to assist me?" Mr. Maingot asked.

Jubilant, more at the prospect of meeting the guru of abdominal operations—my hero—than the prospect of the appendectomy, I headed home to our flat in Albany Street in the dark of London's post-rush hour traffic. Victoria was on duty, so there was no dinner. I made a cup of tea, grabbed a scone, and pulled Mr. Maingot's well-worn book, *Abdominal Operations,* off the shelf. I started to reread Chapter 52, "The Treatment of Acute Appendicitis," with its step-by-step instructions and accompanying line diagrams of the operation. The stakes were high because this was no longer a theoretical exercise. This was it—the real thing!

I met the great man himself in the surgeon's changing room. He was of medium height, with the paunch of prosperity, and spoke softly yet with authority. He was probably in his early fifties. He thanked me for the referral and said he'd already met the Erdmans and examined Timothy. The boy's history and physical findings were classic. We changed into green scrubs and donned our caps.

As I stood in front of the sink, I glanced through the window and observed that Timothy was already anesthetized and on the operating table. Fluids were running through an intravenous drip into his veins, rehydrating him, and he received a push of antibiotics to help his natural immune system kill off the bacteria infecting his appendix.

The scrub nurse washed his lower abdomen, painted it with an antiseptic, and draped it with sterile green towels, covering the rest of his body with sterile sheets. Mr. Maingot and I stood at the sink lathering up, now wearing masks. Suddenly, he asked, "Would you like to take out the appendix?"

Thrilled, I held the scalpel like the bow of a violin as I had learned when operating on my own patients at the Royal Ear Hospital, grateful to Desmond for teaching me surgical techniques. I proceeded to make a three- to four-inch McBurney's skin incision. Using two retractors, Mr. Maingot pulled back the skin and subcutaneous fat while simultaneously blotting the bleeders. I incised the external oblique muscle, starting a gridiron incision, the very incision I'd had difficulty explaining to Ingrid a few years earlier. Mr. Maingot moved the retractors deeper, carefully stretching the dark red muscle fibers apart, widening the incision. As the deeper layers were incised, the retractors followed, placed deeper and stretching the tissues farther apart. We were like well-rehearsed dancers complementing each other's steps. We did not speak. I merely followed my mental map from Chapter 52, guided by the master surgeon himself.

I stared at the abdominal contents, spellbound by the body's beauty. I wanted to tell the guts that I loved then and that I had missed them. My last glimpse of the abdomen was at Mass General in Boston, a long time ago.

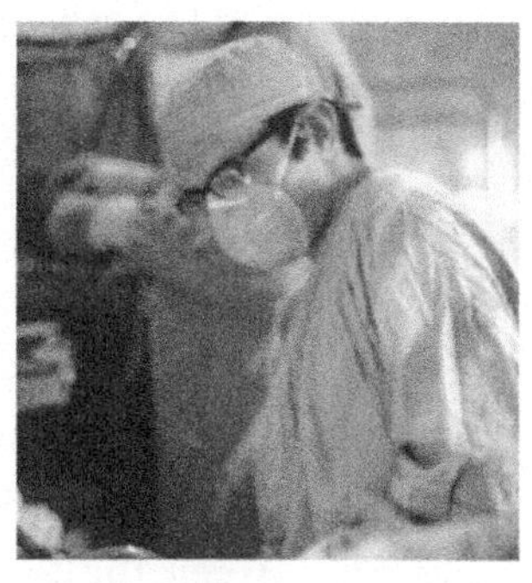

I was nudged out of my reverie by the scrub nurse, who handed me moist gauze lap pads to wall off the coils of the writhing pink and healthy-looking small bowel, isolating the glistening beige caecum and the appendix. Touching the tissues added to my sensuous elation, while operating in my favorite domain gave me an addictive high, one better than sex.

The scrub nurse slapped a Babcock clamp into my palm. It was designed to encircle the appendix without crushing it, as a means to hold it. I applied it around the appendix, which was about two inches long. Its encapsulating blood vessels were inflamed, the tissue infected, and its necrotic tip looked bluish-green and smelled like ripe Gorgonzola. Even so, it was a thing of beauty. I applied a second Babcock clamp. Tugging slightly on both, I cautiously eased the appendix to the center of the open wound and started to free it from its tethered tissues.

I was about to use the Metzenbaum scissors handed to me to sever the tissue when Mr. Maingot interceded.

"Give him a scalpel," he said to the scrub nurse. And to me he said, "You don't cut your steak with scissors, do you? Always use the knife . . . you're a surgeon."

I divided the tissue, completely freeing up the appendix. The operation proceeded in silence, save for the rhythmic beeping of the cardiac monitor. I tied off the proximal cut margins of the mesoappendix with thin silk ligatures while Mr. Maingot released each clamp. With black silk, I placed a purse-string suture in the caecum surrounding the appendix.

Every choreographed move was designed to avoid an inadvertent stab or cut to a team member, thereby preventing the risk of transmitting hepatitis or other blood borne diseases. Keeping my vision focused on the structures, I merely held out my right hand, and the scrub nurse placed a knife into it. I was operating in the lap of luxury. No talk, just hand signals with the scrub knowing exactly what I wanted.

I cut between the two clamps at the base of the appendix and excised it, handing it off to her. Mr. Maingot grunted his approval. Using the electric Bovie knife, he coagulated the stump. The effects of Bovieing leaves broiled, charcoal-looking tissue, and the rising white smoke has the odor of burnt meat.

With forceps, Mr. Maingot dunked the stump into the base of the caecum as I snugged tight the purse string and tied it off before removing the lap pads in the wound. The circulating nurse started to count them, as well as the number of needles used, to ensure none were left in the abdomen.

The anesthetist stared at us over the drape, as if to signal that we were wasting his time, so I proceeded to close the peritoneum. After I tied off the final stitch, Mr. Maingot indicated to the scrub by merely raising his right eyebrow that he wanted to irrigate the wound between each layer. She provided warm sterile saline in a small basin, which he poured into the wound. Bits of white fat and tissue debris floated to the surface. I sucked out the irrigation fluid and debris using the sucker. Mr. Maingot then sponged the wound, again using lap pads. He was averse to using the traditionally provided three by three gauze sponges to avoid the unforgivable sin of accidentally overlooking one inside the patient.

A needle holder with a silk suture was placed in my hand, and Mr. Maingot whispered, "Interrupted sutures," indicating that he wanted the gridiron incision to be closed with non-continuous sutures. As I did this, Mr. Maingot cut above the top of each knot, thus moving the operation along rapidly until I loosely closed the skin. I had performed my first appendectomy to cure a fellow human. I could not think of a greater sacrament that I could contribute to humanity. The appendectomy had been performed thirteen years to the day my appendix was removed in Cairo and fifty years after King George VI had his removed in the very same operating theater at St. George's Hospital. I was overcome with a sense of humility.

Timothy's anesthetic was reduced, and he began to wake up. The anesthetist recorded wound closure time as 9:16 p.m., blood loss as minimal, and a correct sponge count. Mr. Maingot applied a dry sterile dressing to the skin incision, writing on it the date and time, and then proclaimed, "You did that with the alacrity of uprooting a turnip." Did he mean it as a compliment?

Mr. Maingot had formally baptized me: I was an abdominal surgeon, at last. Now, I had to earn my stripes, the primary followed by the fellowship exam. Driving home, I was determined to heal myself and to rid myself of past demons. Little did I suspect the journey that lay ahead.

My first private patient, no doubt, provided Mr. Maingot with a handsome fee. In my euphoria of having done my first appendectomy, I forgot to bill Mr. Erdman for the hotel visit and for an assistant's fee. A few weeks later, a different blue envelope floated through my mail drop. After reading it, I pasted Mr. Maingot's thank you note into his book.

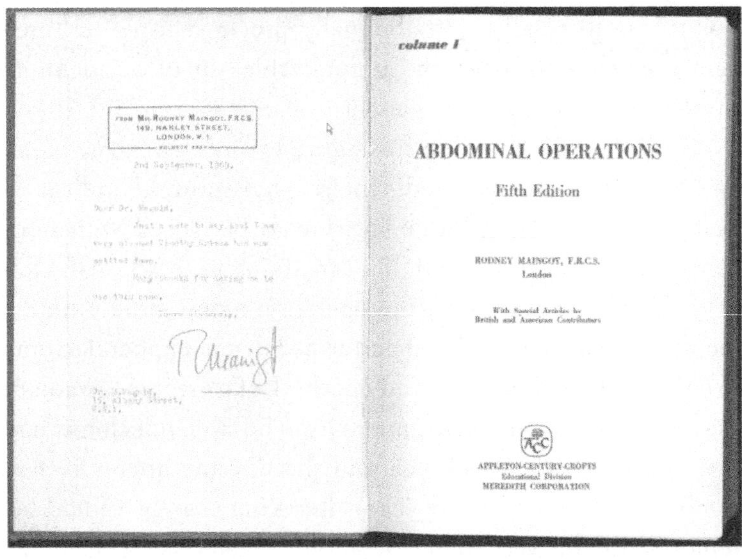

FROM MR. RODNEY MAINGOT, F.R.C.S.
149, HARLEY STREET,
LONDON, W.1

2nd September, 1969.

Dear Dr. Meguid,

[illegible]

volume I

ABDOMINAL OPERATIONS

Fifth Edition

RODNEY MAINGOT, F.R.C.S.
London

With Special Articles by
British and American Contributors

APPLETON-CENTURY-CROFTS
Educational Division
MEREDITH CORPORATION

I was relieved when Dr. B. came back six weeks later on a Friday evening as office hours were winding down. After Jenny said her goodbyes, we sat in his office while he sipped his glass of sherry. "Well, how was it? Jenny said you did well. Ready to join me as a partner?"

I laughed. "I still have my sights set on surgery if I pass the primary fellowship. But I learned a hell of a lot of practical medicine, for which I thank you."

He drove me in his Morris Minor through a drizzle in the dark to our flat in Albany Street. The rhythm of the windshield wipers was the only sound as we both sat lost in our respective thoughts. I was happy to have had the exposure but glad to be relieved from the responsibility of general practice life. It didn't suit me. My aim was to hunker down and study in earnest for the fellowship exam. I had about seven weeks to prepare.

"You wouldn't be interested in working for the ESSO office in Park Lane, would you? You'd see tanker captains two mornings a week for their annual physical. They pay handsomely, £60 per week," and he made a low whistle through his teeth. "It's just for three weeks. Would you?"

"What a temptation! Perhaps another time. Right now, I need to continue to study and prepare myself for the exam, and God knows there are temptations and too many distractions."

He looked over with an inquisitive look. "Well, I'm your GP and your friend. If you need to talk, you know where you can find me." Did he suspect? Had Jenny mentioned to him the occasional calls I got from Hanna? I wondered. He extended his hand, which I shook.

He dropped me off at 15 Albany Street with a wave of his hand as I stepped into the night's rain. Looking up, the lights were not on in our flat. Victoria wasn't home. I missed her already, for I wanted to share my triumph with her.

25

THE COMPLEXITY OF NEED

Every one rushes elsewhere and into the future, because no one wants to face one's own inner self.
—Michel de Montaigne

Blinded by hubris from the recently performed appendectomy and with my wife too entrenched in her world, I called Hanna several days later. I wanted to dance, to express my joy, success and liberation—a relief from the seemingly eternal bookwork.

We met. The strategy of minimal suspicion set in for Hanna: no perfume, no lipstick, no make-up, and no hickeys. For me, I chose only restaurants that were far removed and unlikely to be in the path of people who might know either of us. Was I playing with fire again?

John extended his overseas stay, and the availability of his flat was a godsend. Being Catholic, Hanna didn't feel comfortable with contraception, preferring to depend on the rhythm method. While that would free me from buying condoms and finding hiding places for them, we agreed that it wouldn't do for her to become pregnant. She finally settled on the pill, which I prescribed for her monthly.

The only time I was emotionally free from worries and the burden of deception was when Victoria and I went for a weekend to the Isle of Serenity. When I would tell Hanna that I was busy, a crestfallen expression would cross her beautiful face. Her gloominess didn't last long, for she'd make a mischievous comment like, "Leave my best friend with me," or "I'll tie the Irish flag around it." We'd laugh, and her jovial mood would return. She'd lean over and kiss me on the cheek as if she forgave me.

Back in London, Victoria's absence didn't help. After the weekend I knew I had to resume studying for the exams. In a weary state of boredom and loneliness, I accepted the job with ESSO. I rationalized that if I failed the Primary the first time I might use the £60 per week to pay for the study courses at the college where attendance cost nearly £75.

Twice a week, I took the bus to Park Lane and disembarked outside the ESSO administrative building, arriving shortly before 10 a.m. The secretary showed me an examining room and told me that I'd see four patients. My approach to these patients was different because the meeting was usually a singular event and most patients didn't present with a complaint. Unlike in Dr. B's practice, there was no time limit when seeing each patient. They were happy to chat, which allowed the development of a level of interpersonal comfort and confidence. I was particularly interested in the amount of alcohol consumed because these men bore a tremendous responsibility for their ship, crew and cargo. Other relevant topics included how much they smoked, their dietary habits, their weight history, their sleep patterns, whether they exercised, and how they entertained themselves during the months-long trips at sea. Occasionally, I'd ask them about the risks they faced concerning sexually transmitted diseases, if I sensed their history was leaning in that direction. Of particular concern was the frequency they bought over-the-counter medications like valium, sleeping pills, steroids, or even anti-hypertensive medication in countries like those in the Middle East where prescriptions were not needed.

The secretary directed the first patient into my practice. Captain Wilson had berthed his oil tanker in Southampton and was on shore leave after eight months at sea. Obtaining a social and past medical history was easy despite not having Captain Wilson's prior medical record. During the interview, I faced a dilemma: he confessed that he was on anti-hypertensive medication to control his blood pressure, which he bought through a friend in Hong Kong. Having told me this, he asked for a refill script and my discretion not to record this fact because it might prejudice his lucrative employment and the retirement bonus he expected in a couple of years.

I paused and looked at him. What to do? What to say? Who would be the injured party if this information was to be omitted? "Let me think about it," was my response while I proceeded to examine him.

The physical examination differed from what I did on Dr. B's patients. I had to assure that patients who spent long months at sea and who didn't have rapid access to physicians were safe. I focused on measuring their blood pressure, carefully examining their chests and hearts, their cardiovascular systems, and their prostates—organs vulnerable to disease in middle-aged, relatively sedentary men. Finally, I'd check them for hernias, which could become troublesome during long voyages.

A nurse drew blood to test routine metabolic, hematological, and lipid profiles and performed an electrocardiogram—an electrical profile of the heart's function—and finally ordered a chest X-ray. The blood would be sent out, and I'd have to request the results before the patient's next visit. However, I could read the EKG and assure myself that the old ticker was functioning well at that moment.

With these normal data in hand, I returned to Captain Wilson to focus on his initial request. He must have seen a young man frowning pensively, searching for the right approach to a delicate question. "Regarding your anti-hypertensive medication, what would you do if you were in my position?"

He grimaced and shifted in his seat, weighing me up. I asked, "Do you know if ESSO would retire you if they know that you were taking high blood pressure pills that you bought on your own? Or would the issue be that you were hiding this information while inadvertently increasing their liability?"

He moved his head from side to side, like a cobra, while considering my remarks.

"I think you would be in a solid legal position if they knew. Afterall this is why they give you annual checkups. My advice is that you stop the contraband medication. I will prescribe the drug and make a note that you are functioning well. I am sure no untoward effect such as a tanker accident will occur. At the most, the company will do a physical on you more frequently."

He seemed pleased with this commonsense approach and gladly departed after his hour-long visit. Three more patients waited for me. I felt glad with what I considered concierge medical care, although I worried that having assured the company that he was fine, he could step out of the office and drop dead from a sudden massive heart attack or, worse, a debilitating stroke. The uncertainty and the haunting anxiety of shift-working for ESSO challenged me.

Victoria was a house officer—an intern. I knew from my own experience the previous year how busy she would be. On the occasional night that she'd come home, she'd want a hot bath to unwind, a meal, maybe do some reading in preparation for a next day conference, and then crash in bed to catch up on lost sleep. Fatigue dowsed arousal and killed libido such that sex was not a priority. It was a distant second—our differences cause distress, for as John Berger said to be desired is perhaps the closest anybody in this life can reach to feeling immortal.

It was wonderful having my wife at home, running a bath for her, preparing dinner and enjoying her presence—her company, her chatter. She never talked about her work, her patients, what she had experienced in the past forty-eight hours and my questions seemed to burden her, rather than open her up. I began to feel unhappy—in a remorseful mood. I was at home alone every day and most nights in our tiny flat. Sitting in front of dry anatomy, physiology and pathology books was hardly inspiring. I was bored and too overwhelmed by loneliness to study for the surgical—the next huge landmark in my life. Loneliness was my acute pain, the albatross I lived with along with my unfulfilled need to be loved—emotions I desperately wanted to expunge.

Frequently, my thoughts drifted to wanting Hanna's company, despite my desperate desire to end our affair. I hesitated calling; I repeatedly reminded myself Victoria was my only love, my true love, my wife, my future, the woman who would bear my children. I believed it in my heart and desperately wanted to be faithful and loyal to her.

In this struggle of consciousness between the taboo of Hanna's tug and my obligations, the want for love won out. I called Hanna on the communal telephone on the landing of the nursing residents at the hospital. If an unknown voice answered, my awkward impulse was to hang up, all the while my heart racing and my palms sweating. When I'd call later, mustering all my courage, I'd request to speak to Hanna in a clipped pseudo-business voice or at other times leave a coded or vague message with the answering voice, presumably a nurse who might recognize me. "Please ask Hanna to telephone

Dr. Meguid. It concerns Mrs. Jones." Both deeds were accompanied with a galloping heart, a dry mouth, a lot of sweating, and the dread of certain gossip about us.

From time to time, a friendly and pleasing voice would volunteer that Hanna had gone out for the evening, saying, "She won't be back till late." Immediately, my burning jealousy for her faithlessness and her neglect made me loathe her. I hoped that my disappointment was recognized over the phone. I'd swear quietly at her adulterous behavior and imagine she was in bed with another man—thoughts that tortured me.

My presumption of her promiscuity angered me and led me to call her an unfaithful harlot in my mind and swear I'd stop seeing her. The irony and irrationality of my response did not elude me. Foolishly, I called again. She answered the phone. In a quiet voice, for fear of being overheard by someone, I suggested we meet early in the morning at Westminster Pier and take a Thames Riverboat to Hampton Court. The weatherman predicted a clear sky, a few clouds, and sunshine.

Fearing the danger of being recognized heightened my nervousness, but seeing her was most agreeable. She was beaming with delight. Her smile and joy lifted my heart and dissipated the dark thoughts and my gnawing loneliness as fast as a cloud passing overhead on a windy day. We sat on the upper deck of the riverboat, taking in the changing scenery as we headed north toward Henley on our three-hour trip: Parliament, leafy suburbia, bombed-out lots, decaying industrial lots, the bridges, the locks, traveling along the course of my previous Thames boat race and getting our fill of sunshine. We sat mostly in silent stillness, my arm occasionally about her shoulder when the wind made her shiver. I wondered what she was thinking about, but did not want to ask, fearing to disturb the harmony and wanting to avoid the touchy aspects of our relationship, that of our mutual jealousy roused by awkward questions—hers, "Do you sleep with your wife?" and mine,

"Where and with whom do you go out at night?" In its place, looks and glances and internal dialogue filled our amity. I drew her close to steal kisses. "One day, I'd love to go to Ireland and meet you there."

"I'll probably be living here. So, don't bother."

Since Hanna was on evening duty starting at 3 p.m., we didn't linger at Hampton Court or buy a souvenir to capture our moment of bliss and sanity. We took the fast train back to London. She must have wondered what was in store for our relationship, for when we parted, I vaguely promised I'd contact her again.

26

THE ADDICTION OF ECSTASY

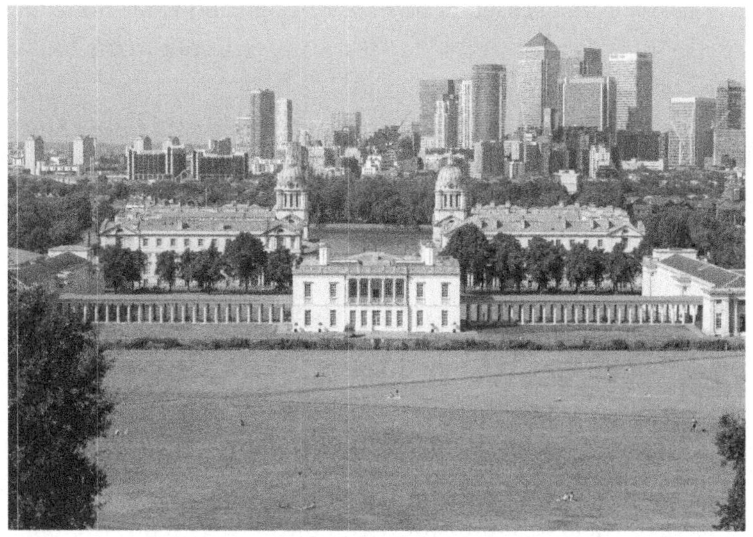

To have her here in bed with me, breathing on me, her hair in my mouth—I count that something of a miracle.

—Henry Miller

Mother was many months-long abroad, either in Germany or Egypt. I couldn't keep track of her movements, not that I cared much, and her infrequent letters were typed single space on both sides of a sheet of airmail paper. They usually announced her past travel and her next destination, but they were too long, and contained gossip or things she wanted me to do for her in Egypt.

Mother had set up a bedroom that she insisted was for my use, failing to accept that Victoria and I were married and we had our own home—that I had cut the cord between us when she abandoned me years ago. Perhaps arranging a room for me was her subconscious wish to have me back, so I would call her "Mutti" or "my mother" instead of the cold noun I used for her —Mother. I had ceased to be hers long ago and I was not going to use the room she had set up for me, at least not in the role of "her son."

Long weekends without Victoria were my soul killer. She'd be on call in the hospital. When I tired of studying at Albany Street, I'd break the monotony and drudgery by taking my books and revision schedule to Mother's flat where I studied. The table in "my bedroom" brimmed with notes, open books and spent cups of coffee.

I'd persuade Hanna to visit me when I was driven by the hunger for her closeness and the momentary need of the security of her embrace, the reassurance that she and I could be alive in my dreary world of study. We met in Greenwich Park near Blackheath. It was a district I was sure provided anonymity. Its gently tumbling hills provided panoramic views overlooking the Old Royal Naval College, Greenwich Hospital and, on the opposite embankment of the Thames, the city of London and Canary Wharf.

We would amble through the grove of ancient chestnut trees on late mornings as the mist rose from the grass into their canopies. Since there were no leash laws, dogs ran about, ignoring their owners' calls when chasing squirrels or the occasional deer. Like the dogs, I felt free of the leash constraint imposed by marriage and welcomed the pleasure of escaping my duty to study. Eventually, we'd make our way out of the walled park to Mother's nearby flat.

Hanna and I settled in Mother's kitchen and drank tea, mainly in silence looking at one another trying to read each other's minds. Our sexual tension rose as our tea cooled. By afternoon, we drifted into that room, where in the gentle tide of love I'd touch her hair, her face, her neck as we slowly stripped each other. She quivered as we removed item by item, to the notes of expressed pleasure and approval enhanced by passionate kisses, exploring tongues, and fumbling fingers—for we could never get enough.

We enjoyed our slow appreciation of seeing and smelling us. My hands stray knowing we'd reach ecstasy. We were connected, our bodies tasted of one another, and we breathed in unison. We lay together, exhausted, both of us wanting time to stop—wanting it to last for eternity.

Resting, my mind drifted to Captain Wilson and his medication. "Can you imagine he wanted me to conspire with him to deceive ESSO about his illicitly taking medications for fear it might prejudice his future? How mendacious of him."

Hanna turned to me, propped up on her elbow, her breasts weighing down against me, "And . . . did you?"

"Of course not. That's being deceitful. Suppose he has a seizure or a TIA (transient ischemic event) leading to an accident where oil would gush out of his tanker and pollute the sea. What a disaster! Can you imagine the upshots when his dishonesty was discovered? And I'd be in cahoots with him?"

"So . . . what happened?"

"Well, I told him I couldn't do it. He should face reality and be honest because the consequences of not doing so had serious outcomes. He would be cheating the company."

She lay down again, eyes fixed forward, and after a silent while she said, "It's like you, really. You're the captain, and I'm the tanker full of your semen." Now, it was I who propped my head on my elbow and looked at her inquisitively.

"Isn't it the same?" she added in a serious voice, glancing at me.

The word adultery crossed my mind. This obsession was an illness—a cancer. Give me a knife so I can cut out this haunting addiction.

27

THE TERROR OF FAILURE

The greatest barrier to success is the fear of failure.
—Sven Eriksson

I faced the written primary surgical fellowship exam with trepidation. Passing it would indicate to the surgical world that my specialty was surgery, and after passing it, I would be eligible for surgical registrar jobs. Seventeen months previously, I had sat for the Licentiate of the Society of Apothecaries examination where, in a matter of several hours, I had poured out five years of accumulated medical knowledge gained in medical school at University College Hospital into blue-covered answering books. I passed this examination. Passing earned me a license to practice medicine in the UK. A few weeks later, my quest to attain the academically acclaimed and more important degree of MBBS was less satisfying; the tension to pass the definitive General Medical Council's qualifying examinations was less urgent, and my desire to purge myself of my accrued learning was less pressing and more tedious. Yet, passing the Medical Council's qualifying exam, I was rewarded with the title "doctor." In both exams, I had a sense of confidence that I knew the information—the medical school curriculum—from which the examination questions would be asked.

The Primary Examination drew from no such set curriculum. The morning of the examination I woke up early to the smell of bacon. Victoria made me a smack-up breakfast along with my favorite tea. She, too, had passed the essential requisite medical degree exam and was making plans to pursue a career in pediatrics.

"This is to fortify you." She must have sensed my tension and reassuringly urged, "Read the questions carefully. Sketch an outline of your answer and then proceed to write." I nodded as I ate my eggs and bacon. "You've been studying for months. I'm sure you'll do fine." She paused before adding, "You always do."

I wish she had not said that. If she only knew how I had been attending to other parts of my brain and body. I had short-changed my studies—the painful deception of a parallel life. I felt awful. Looking up, I saw her external beauty and all the virtues I had admired and overlooked for the past months. All the virtues which had made me fall in love with her. At that moment I didn't deserve her, nor did I deserve to be rewarded with passing the exam.

In the grand scheme of things, I could say that I had studied. Yet I didn't feel prepared, not enough to assuage my sense of apprehension—the terror of failure was ingrained into my DNA inherited from my father and a long line of Sa'idi's in Upper Egypt. Had I covered the fields of anatomy, physiology and surgical pathology appropriately? My fear of failure, along with the distraction of covering Dr. B's general practice for six weeks, a stint working as a physician for ESSO, plus my inability to find and review past primary surgical fellowship exam papers, added up to a profound lack of confidence.

But the major factor in this brew was my off and on attention to Hanna instead of my studies. I had become addicted to her because she accepted me, made me feel alive but above all she awakened my feelings again—feelings I had buried to protect myself from pain. I sensed that her acceptance of me related to the feeling of us being "the other," that which Dr. Rosenheim spelled out and Victoria couldn't see.

Loaded with this baggage, I walked briskly through a cool morning to the front entrance of the Examination Hall Queen Square in Old Gloucester Street—as if heading to an abattoir. A beadle barked at me, "Candidates enter the examination hall via a basement door," and he redirected me around the building to a narrow back street.

There, Mr. Palmer, a formidable army type in a smart mauve frock coat, directed me to a murmur-filled hall with examination desks. I recognized no one as I took my seat. Face down in front of me lay a white sheet of paper and a blue examination booklet.

The anatomy questions were obscure, nuanced, and I could barely understand them. By asking *this* question about *that* anatomical structure, I wondered *what* answer they were seeking. I answered as best as I could, hardly satisfied.

I moved to the physiology paper. I found the questions difficult to understand. My answers became convoluted and meandering in the hope of befuddling the examiner. Both in the written essay and the orals questions, I wasn't on the examiner's wave length—we didn't click. Matters didn't improve with the pathology questions. I was a driver careening down the road with no control of my car, heading for a crash.

Two days later, I faced the dreaded *viva voce*—the orals, with four different examiners who could quiz me about any aspect of surgical anatomy, histology, physiology and pathology. From the very beginning, my composure, demeanor, even my posture, reflected my lack of self-confidence. Sitting in front of my two surgical anatomy inquisitors, I waffled my way through the examinations, my answers lacking conviction. It was painful to hear myself. My strategy was to prevent the examiner from asking another question by talking endlessly because I knew, for sure, I wouldn't know how to answer their next question. I felt a real fraud for bluffing my way into a profession whose standard I knew I had not earned and did not deserve. When it came to their interrogation of physiology, I wanted to melt away in my chair.

I could barely look the last two surgeons in the eyes. The first asked, "What is a sphincter? And give me some examples."

I heard myself say, "What do you mean by sphincter, sir? I don't understand the question." What was there not to understand? Where was my mind? The first surgeon impaled me on his examiner's sword of questions, while the second finished any prospect of my passing by skewering me with my ignorance. Both watched me metaphorically crumble and bleed to death.

By midday, cross-examinations in all topics had concluded. We were advised by Mr. Palmer, in his booming voice, that the examiners first have their customary traditional three-course lunch that was served by elderly helpers, preceded by a glass of sherry and concluded with a selection of delectable cheeses and crackers with a glass of port. And, only following lunch, would Mr. Palmer announce the numbers that indicated the names of those who had earned the honor of an elevated status —"The three Ps that deservedly placed a candidate onto the first rung of the ladder to 'power, prestige and pocketbook,'"— as he phrased it, to "righteous membership in the profession of barber surgeon."

I retreated to The Swan, which was a few minutes from the examination hall and open for lunch. Several other candidates had congregated there, and together, we commiserated, drawn by the certainty of having done poorly but longing for some glimmer of hope in our gloom. I sat among the other candidates, nursing half a pint of lemonade shandy and licking my self-inflicted wounds—more attention to Hanna than to my books. The mood among my fellow candidates swung from foul to fouler to desperate, like a dark and hopeless plot in a Kafka novel. I heaped all sorts of punishing and self-deprecating names on myself, castigated myself for ill-preparedness, squandered energy, obsession with another woman and my deceitful behavior. I hated myself. Sitting in this stew of self-made shit, I waited in agony for the four o'clock congregation at the examination hall with Mr. Palmer. It was like waiting for the hangman, I imagined.

He boomed out successful candidates by number. Unperturbed by the howls from failed candidates, Mr. Palmer continued down the list to pronounce with gusto the number of successful candidates, all of whom exited via the front door, eyes averted, leaving behind their failed and bleeding colleagues. When he called a number after mine, I knew I had failed, as I had feared, as I suspected. I was among the contemptible eighty percent who did not satisfy the examiners—the dross, the unworthy, the undesirable, the disreputable, the despicable of surgically aspiring degenerates.

The failed candidates departed via the basement door through which they had entered. I joined a group of disappointed wretches who wanted to express their misdirected frustration and anger at failing. As we ambled together along the outside of the back of Queen Hall, talk of disappointment at failing and the need for revenge toward the examiners grew. In an act of retaliation, the failed candidates pissed in unison into the ventilation system of the examination hall—ten powerful streams of urine aimed right into the vents.

I limped home to a cold, dark, empty flat and crawled into bed without eating dinner. At least I was alone; Victoria was on duty in the hospital. As I drifted asleep, I had two thoughts. I had to pass this exam if I wanted to become a surgeon and possibly go to America. The next opportunity to sit for this exam would be in June 1970. I resolved to sign up for the courses at the Royal College to better prepare myself for the repeat exam. And second, I was determined to cease my distracting thoughts of Hanna.

ROYAL COLLEGE OF SURGEONS OF ENGLAND

EXAMINATION HALL
8-11, QUEEN SQUARE
LONDON W.C.1

Dr M. Meguid

F.R.C.S.

The Examinations Secretary of the Royal College of Surgeons of England forwards the undermentioned Report of the Examiners upon Candidate No. 173 who failed to satisfy them at the Examination in FEB 1970.

Primary Examination

	Anatomy	Physiology	Pathology
Paper	PASSED	POOR	POOR
Oral		POOR	FAIR

Final Examination

Paper

Clinical

Operations and Surgical Anatomy

Pathology

The pass grade is "Fair"
Other grades: "Poor," "Very Poor," "Bad"

Checked by

This information is available only in the case of unsuccessful Candidates.

28

DAMNATION OF DESIRE

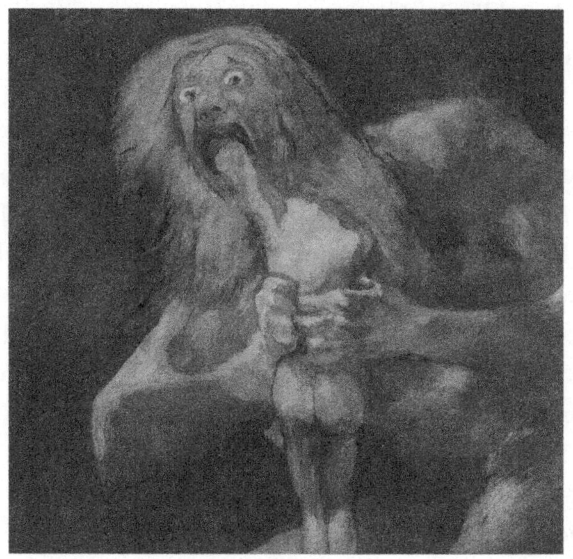

Saturn Devouring His Son, Goya

All sins tend to be addictive,
And the terminal point of addiction is damnation.
—W.H. Auden

My attempts to stop seeing Hanna were futile. So, when she suddenly told me that she was going to visit her family in County Tyrone, I felt she was trying to put space and distance between us. She mentioned that she wasn't sure she would come back. And as if to bring a point home, she said, "I might try and get a job as a Sister on the medical ward or outpatient clinic of the local hospital." Listening to her plans, I realized that I would miss her.

My relationship with Hanna was getting out of hand, especially when she continued to ask if I slept with my wife. I loved Victoria but desired Hanna. I had no thoughts of leaving my wife, and Hanna knew this. Perhaps, she was trying to end the relationship. When Hanna returned, if she returned, I resolved to end the addiction I had for her.

I welcomed the time for my exam preparations. I would be forced to face my books and surgical notes while struggling to get her image out of my mind. Given my fractured past, Victoria provided stability and status. I was proud of her and proud to be with her. I loved her. That's the relationship I knew I should be working on. I focused on my studies and Victoria when she was available.

Victoria and I returned from the Agra after seeing the latest James Bond movie in Leicester Square on a Friday evening, and as we entered the flat, the phone rang. "Darling, can you take that?" Victoria said as she rushed to the loo. "It may be the hospital . . . but I absolutely must have a pee."

I picked up the receiver, wondering who'd be calling so late in the evening.

"Jesus. Where have you been? I've been calling you all evening," I heard Hanna's irritated voice. She had been drinking with the girls and was calling from a coin box in a pub. I was startled; Hanna had never called me at home before.

I heard Victoria flush the toilet and start to wash her hands.

"Are you back?" I said, rapidly cupping the mouthpiece.

"No, Jesus. I'm on the moon. Where do you think I am?" came her Irish drawl. "I've got to see you . . ."

"I'm busy this weekend," I half-whispered. "Meet me Monday evening."

"No, damn you, it's important," she said, adding, "I've got to see you . . . tomorrow . . ."

Victoria came out of the bathroom and headed for me. "Who is it darling?"

Raising my voice while turning away from Victoria I said, "Yes, Mr. Maingot, I'll be there."

"Holy Mother Mary. What's with this Maingot crap?" came the Irish lilt, "Four o'clock at the gazebo in Regent's Park. Don't be late, it's important," she added again.

"That will be fine, Mr. Maingot, four o'clock tomorrow, I'll be there," I emphasized to ensure Victoria had heard, and I hung up. My heart was racing in the pit of my stomach.

"What is it darling? You haven't forgotten, have you? We're going down to the Isle of Wight tomorrow." She seemed perplexed.

"Mr. Maingot wants me to assist him on a private patient . . . quite an honor."

"What? Tomorrow? On my weekend off? I get so few as house officer."

"Yes, it's one of his patients that he admitted to a clinic in Harley Street. Wants to do something or other in her belly, I couldn't quite follow . . ."

"At four in the afternoon?"

"Well, he probably couldn't get an earlier start time. I don't know how long I'll be," I added.

"Can't he find someone else to assist him? Now, it looks you'll have to miss my friends, who all will be there." After a pause, she added in a less whiny voice, "Darling, do phone him back and let him know. I'm sure he'll understand and find someone else. Anyway, how much is he paying you?"

"Look, I can't do that. He wouldn't have phoned me if it weren't important, and he needed my help. Can't you see? I suggest you take the train down, and stay as long as you like. I'm sure Shirley will understand."

"Well, this has thoroughly spoiled a nice evening," Victoria said in a huff. "I'm going to bed."

I felt like a prick. Why hadn't Hanna suggested 9 a.m., and what was so important that it couldn't wait? Why so late? Was she working the morning shift? Hanna had probably found a job back home, or had she met someone else? Had her father, a diabetic, had a stroke, or what? I lay awake next to Victoria.

I accompanied my wife to Waterloo Station to catch the 9:03 a.m. "You'll have to get yourself something to eat. I didn't shop since we were going to Mummy's," she told me.

I nodded. "I'll probably have lunch in the hospital cafeteria. Don't worry about me, just enjoy yourself and give them all my apologies," I said.

This time I bought flowers for her mother and a rose for her by way of expressing my sincere love and apologies. The flowers made me feel less guilty. I gave her a peck on the offered cheek—a gesture not reassuringly intimate. She briefly hung out of the window as the train pulled out of Waterloo, and I waved at her diminishing image, as if to ensure she had gone.

I darted into the nearest telephone kiosk. It reeked of smoke and urine. I dialed Hanna's number. The line was busy. Impatiently, I tried again, but it was still busy. In my mind's eye, I could imagine the common phone box in the corridor of the nurse's dormitory, the one I'd never seen, probably with a queue of nurses lining up to call family, friends, and lovers—a weekend ritual cemented by custom and cheaper telephone rates. It was still busy when I tried once more, so I slammed down the receiver, recovered my coins, and realized why men peed in the booth—a frustrated piss.

Should I just take the Tube to her hospital and try to see her? After her long absence, I felt the urge, a wanting in my bones, one I recognized that spelled intimacy. This was a futile idea. She might be on the ward or attending mass at Holy Cross. The day dragged on. I read the newspaper, unable to stomach my surgical texts.

I went early to Regent's Park and stood by the gazebo, hoping she'd appear sooner. The Coldstream Guard band played tunes from *My Fair Lady* in the bright London Indian summer. In my mind's eye, I could see her hazel-green eyes, playful and inviting, and her loosely slung breasts swaying as she approached me, as I had seen so many times before—sights I enjoyed. Time passed. And passed. Had she forgotten?

My face lit up, seeing her walking stridently along the path. We approached each other, I in slow motion, and she like a bullet. I wanted to kiss her but she averted her face, presenting her cheek. Oh no. Another cheek! She always kissed on the lips. Something was amiss. Hanna seemed cold, more guarded. She stepped back and looked at me. I waited.

"Oh, God. It's great to see you," I said. "I missed you so much. How was your trip home? Tell me all about it." I took her hand and steered her to an empty park bench in the shade of a huge willow tree. She paused, looked at me, scooted a few feet away from me, and stated plainly, "I think I'm pregnant."

"You *think*?"

"Christ . . . I just missed my second period."

"Aren't you panicking? You're on the pill," I said incredulously. "How could that happen when you've been taking the pill regularly?"

"Yeah, every fucking morning, despite them making me queasy." She was angry.

"Better safe than sorry."

"Well, it didn't work, did it? I took it every fucking morning for four months just because you wanted me to . . . except . . ." and she hesitated. "I stopped taking it."

"What? The pill? Why?"

"My mother would kill me if she discovered them. She's a devout Catholic. My father would kill you," and sniffing, she added, "well, both of us. My siblings would probably disown me, too."

I felt my blood pressure rising. How could she stop taking the pills without involving me or at least mentioning it? Was this a trap to rope me into marriage? Both of us had too much to lose.

She had come alone to England four years ago to educate herself and raise her station in life. She had ventured into the cosmopolitan world of London, overcoming educational obstacles to become a successful staff nurse with the ambition of becoming a ward Sister, perhaps even a Matron.

Silence followed as I tried to work out the possible timing of her pregnancy. "You were gone longer . . . more like three weeks."

"No, I wasn't. Just over two."

"Could it be another man? I mean, in Ireland? An old boyfriend, or a new flame?" The second I uttered these words I regretted them, for a hurtful look of profound disbelief flooded her face.

"Holy Mother Mary . . ."

I covered my face with my hands, and then, I embraced her.

"I'm sorry. Really sorry for saying or even thinking that and hurting you." She wept, nuzzled into my shoulder. In the numbed silence that engulfed us, I felt my world slip into a dark void of disbelief, denial and suspicion. In the maelstrom of guilt and confusion, I felt a dull ache arising in the pit of my stomach with the seismic reality of my responsibility. Her sobs abated. Leaning away, she took my pocket square to wipe the mascara off her cheeks.

"What should we do?" I asked tentatively, thinking partly aloud. I shifted. Uneasy. I looked at her sideways, trying to assess the veracity of this very appealing young woman's denial. Was she telling me the truth? She held her gaze on the grass in front of her. "Have you been late before?"

"No. I've been like clockwork, every four weeks since I was thirteen."

"I've heard that in all the pregnant young Irish girls who came by themselves and that I delivered during obstetrics," I said quietly, wondering where the truth lay. Speaking up, I said, "Maybe it's just late, then . . . the excitement of going home, demands of travel and stress . . ."

"Holy Mother Mary. Sick to my stomach for the last three mornings. I went out this morning and bought a pregnancy test kit from Boots."

"You did? And?"

"It's positive," she said in a low voice, as if passersby might hear.

"Did you follow the instructions precisely?"

"Holy Mother Mary . . ."

"How come then? I mean, how did this happen? You're sure?"

How powerful denial can be in the face of an unexpected and terrible complication.

"Jesus wept . . . No, I'm just imagining it. It's all a game. What do you think you, asshole?" she said sarcastically. She was irate and looked away. I watched the band rearranging their sheet music, preparing to play another tune.

"Have you told anyone? And have you thought what you'll want to do?" No response. She turned to me again as I moved closer to her.

We sat in silence, each lost in our own thoughts.

Hanna wouldn't be able to continue working at Bethnal Green once the pregnancy showed. Such was society's shame—particularly in her community for a pregnant, unmarried woman in those days. I imagine it would have been the same in Egypt. Sheikh Amin took in—adopted—Abu Sabour's daughter from Alexandria. Here in England or back home there was Catholic Charities who would take the child.

What were her options? I imagined that she would not want to return to her family in Ireland in this state. If she went through with the pregnancy and had a child, she would face a life of gossip and disgrace, and I doubt her mother would help in child rearing. The stigma would isolate her, perhaps even the entire family, from the tight-knit Catholic Church and her community. If they objected to her being on the pill, then I doubt they would welcome her with open arms, pregnant and unwed. They might send her to a Magdalene Laundry for fallen women or a convent to have the child. Silence descended on us as we both were lost in our own world.

Staring at her shoes, she said in a quiet sorrowful voice, "There was a girl in my class. Margaret was her name. She got banged-up by one of the boys. We were sixteen. None of the lads owned up. She entered a Magdalene charity home. They took her son away from her after two days. They said for adoption. She's still there. No one has seen her again. It's been many years. I doubt she'll ever come out." She now looked at me.

I liked the idea of having a child, but could I really cope with an infant right now, and what would I tell Victoria? I felt deeply remorseful. The male side of the of this issue had become really personal—yet again. Trapped, I was accountable . . . my responsibility.

I weighed up separating from Victoria. I could not envision leaving her. During Victoria's constant absence I had filled the void by inviting Hanna into my life and in the process, I betrayed Victoria—betrayed all of us. I became lonely. The past demons of childhood of having no one near left me afraid of being alone—I needed the security of close comfort—as Oma had provided me in the years of Mother's absence.

"These kits are new, and no one knows how reliable they are. I think you should see a doctor to confirm your suspicions. Then, we can talk again about our options once we know for sure."

"I followed instructions, asshole. Anyway, I *know* my body, and I am sure. What solution do you have in mind?"

"Would you want this child?"

"Holy Mother Mary . . ."

I took that to mean no. The solution and responsibility now lay totally with me. "I see." After a moment's hesitation, I continued, "I know of someone in Harley Street who could help us. She would take care of things quietly; she's one of us, no fuss, no charge. Nobody would know. You'd be right as rain again."

She stared at me, slowly nodded in agreement, and rose. "It's the best thing," she whispered. "I've got to get going." She walked away at an unhurried pace, not waiting, away from the band, away from *My Fair Lady,* away from me, away from the tumult of emotions. I gazed after her, unsure of what might transpire. Would she go if I made the arrangements?

I ran after her. "I'll phone you, tomorrow evening, with some news."

"I'd like to believe you," she said over her shoulder, increasing her pace.

That was painful to hear.

I contacted Desmond, and within a couple of hours, he gave me clear instruction as to where to go near Harley Street on Tuesday afternoon at 2 p.m. If Victoria found out, or if I went with my tail between my legs and told her of the situation, she would be devastated—trust shattered. Would she understand my explanation that I didn't do it to wound her? That I did it from my innate sense of insecurity and vanity?

I met Hanna again with the news. We went to the Rose Garden's Tea House. Sitting at a small table discretely placed out of the main traffic, we had our tea in silence in the late afternoon sun—scones, clotted cream, raspberry jam and her favorite Earl Gray tea. Simon and Garfunkel's song "Bridge over Troubled Water" wafted over the air from a transistor. I handed her Desmond's note and went over the instructions: Tuesday. Eat a light breakfast. No lunch. At the clinic, ask for Elizabeth. Present this note. She'll help you register. Hanna nodded. There followed an awkward silence.

I wondered what would happen if I went with her.

It wasn't customary in the 1960s for men to be involved with female issues of this nature, or even to have them observe or participate in childbirth. So, Hanna's answer didn't surprise me when I asked if she wanted me to go with her.

"Oh, God no. No. You'd embarrass me. Anyway, they wouldn't want you there."

I had seen a string of young, pregnant American women every Tuesday morning in Dr. B's GP office. I'd attest that they were pregnant and send them on to Harley Street. The following morning, I'd see them again to make sure they were fit to fly back to the United States. Magdalena, the American women, even the senator's daughter had done physiologically well. What the emotional damage was remained unseen by me, unreported and often buried. "You haven't changed your mind about next Tuesday, have you?"

"Oh, no. Jesus . . . no! I don't think you're ready to become a father or leave your wife." This set me back, for she had never asked me to, but she was right. Yet she never tested her assumptions.

The waitress came. We rose, I paid, and we left. I held Hanna's hand and took her to the Tube along empty Sunday streets in the fading afternoon light. I bought her ticket back to the hospital, kissed the presented cheek. No mouth kisses. She lingered, searching my eyes. I wished I knew how to span the gulf between us, how to reach out, touch her, heal her, say I was sorry, truly, truly sorry. She turned and passed through the turnstile, stepped onto the down escalator, and didn't look back. She disappeared into the subterranean world, out of my sight. My heart ached—for her and my transgressions.

PART V

LONDON

SPRING TO SUMMER 1970

Mourning is the price we pay for having the courage to love others.
—Irvin D. Yalom MD

29

POSTMORTEM

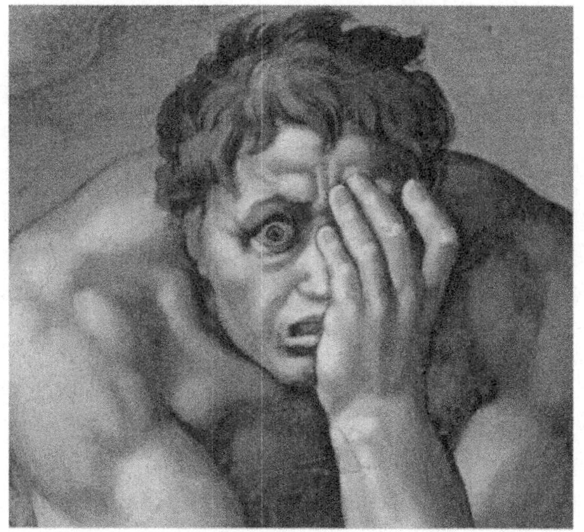

Last Judgement, Michelangelo

Maybe all one can do is hope to end up with the right regrets.
—Arthur Miller

There was no hole on this earth deep or dark enough for me to crawl into and hide. My confusions about sex had repeatedly echoed in intimate situations during my childhood and into adulthood.

If Victoria suspected my infidelity, she didn't make it known, but I doubted she knew.

I could not resist Hanna's flattery and flirtations in my egotistic sense of loneliness and insecurity and as a result of my unresolved anger at Mother. Lonesome for Victoria, I allowed Hanna into my life. She filled the void of longing until it grew into a madness for her. I had rationalized that I was giving Victoria the room she needed to complete her medical studies to become a physician. In reality, I had deceived them both, and by doing so, I had cheated us all.

Back at my desk, I could not stop ruminating and trying to make sense of the situation with Hanna. Should I have objected to her solution? Was it the right thing to do? Did we have this right? Would we be snuffing out a potential daughter or a son, or simply removing a bloody clump of cells? What if Hanna died from an anesthetic mishap like I'd witnessed twice last year? No, I reasoned with myself, this was a private clinic, where others had gone and done well. *Let matters run their course*, I thought. My brooding made me realize I was glad she wanted to get it behind her. Though I was thankful Mother hadn't made the same choice.

Until this unfortunate event, my entire existence had been focused on the accumulation, implementation and practice of my clinical skills—to help patients, to better their lot and to heal them. My purpose in life was to cure and lift the human spirit. I wished that its soul would be well cared for although I wasn't sure if the soul lay in the scientific realm or in the spiritual one. Nevertheless, I prayed for it, Hanna and us.

A week after, Hanna and I met for lunch in a dim pub basement near Bethnal Green Hospital. She wore her normal cheery affect, although underneath the façade, she was more subdued than usual, and we both had perfunctory smiles. It was her day off, and things had profoundly changed. She now wore make-up, perfume, lipstick, and an emerald ring. I got the message—a new beginning for her. We both spoke little and merely picked at our sandwiches, a novelty in pubs at the time, and sipped our drinks.

"How are you? How do you feel?

"Right as rain. Elizabeth is such a kind lady."

There wasn't much news to share. The amorous fling had run its course, and where there once was passion and the invincibility of love, there sat only two wounded humans dealing with hurt, anguish and regret—at many different levels. The loving words had been spoken. The kindness, company, and comfort extended to each other had evaporated. All that remained was mutual empathy. As we negotiated the terms of our parting in silence, as if we could read each other's minds, she passed me a slip of paper. The poem scripted in her hand read:

Remember me when this you see,
Remember me forever,
Remember the good times,
We had in 212 together.

"Thank you. How can I ever forget you? You hold a special place in my heart. I'll be sure to keep it." She maintained her mirthful visage betrayed only by her sad eyes.

I slid my hand across the table to squeeze hers. "No matter your belief," I said, "God is merciful," I murmured softly. It could have been the epitaph placed on the tombstone of our affair.

With that, we parted.

30

PROMISE OF SUNSHINE

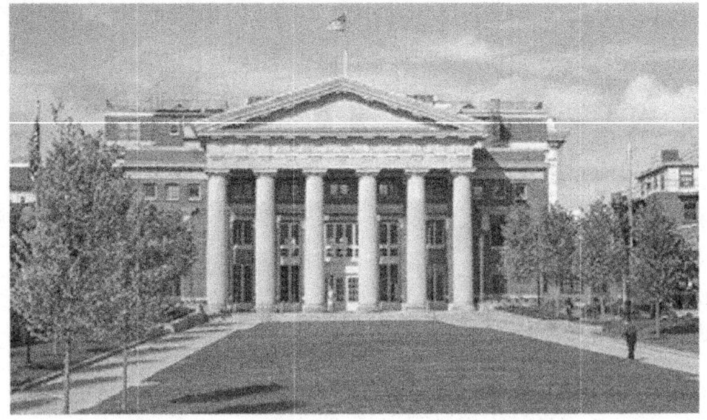

Courtesy Brigham and Women's Hospital

Trouble lies in sullen pools along the road I've taken
Sightless windows stare the empty street
No love beckons me save that which I've forsaken
The anguish of my solitude is sweet.
—Robert Mitchum

Eighteen months earlier when in the United States, I had interviewed for surgical training in Boston and New York before returning to London. I had received two definitive offers. Dr. Francis Moore, in Boston, had offered me a position as a second-year resident in general surgery starting July 1, 1970.

HARVARD MEDICAL SCHOOL

DEPARTMENT OF SURGERY

FRANCIS D. MOORE, M.D.
Moseley Professor of Surgery

Peter Bent Brigham Hospital
721 Huntington Avenue
Boston, Massachusetts 02115
Telephone 617 - [illegible]

April 2, 1969

Dr. Marwan Meguid
15 Albany Street
Regent's Park
London, N.W.1., England

Dear Dr. Meguid:

Thank you very much for your note.

When I wrote you in February about an interview, it had quite slipped my mind that we had a chance to talk together on the 8th of December, 1967.

We are looking forward to having you here with us and we can offer you a position in July of 1970.

I do not need anymore interviews, but what I do need is your completed application form together with a photograph of yourself and the names of two or three people to whom I may write for additional references.

When we get this paper work tidied up, then we can focus more clearly on the precise level of residency training at which you should enter our system, and precisely how long a time of training we should offer you at this time.

It is my understanding that you qualified in April, [illegible]. This would suggest to me that if you come to join us in 1970, you would be a candidate for two years of Junior Residency.

Let me hear from you on this, and do send me the form and the photograph to help me recall our interview together.

Thank you very much.

Very truly yours,

Francis D. Moore, M.D.

FDM:[illegible]

Enclosure

He had received several letters of reference. I was glad that Drs. Stern, Hart, Gilliland and Kingdom had come through. I was most grateful to all these good souls on both sides of the pond.

The congenial head of the residency program at Roosevelt Hospital had sent a lengthier note, proceeding with some courteous niceties, including a request for two references, and then offering me a general surgical internship as we had discussed in New York.

The news was liberating; I had a potential future in surgery. In America, a community of immigrants, I would not be hampered by my cultural heritage. The energy of the country's "can do" philosophy meant that Camelot lay across the ocean. Could it be that the sun shone over the horizon?

The two letters added to the urgency to succeed at the next exam. This time, failure was not an option.

"Is this what you want?" Victoria asked when we spoke about the letters. The dilemma I faced was which proposal to accept: Boston or New York? The letter from Boston offered a job only for me. The letter from New York recognized that Victoria, too, was a physician and included an offer for her. But New York was not Harvard. The choice would place us on an entirely different career trajectory, an academic one at Harvard versus a private practice pathway in New York.

I visited John Rackey, who thought I was mad to ask. "It's not even a consideration. The average American medical student would give his right ball to get an offer from Harvard." Such a forceful statement from an even-tempered Yale graduate and Air Force pilot cum med student, who was also seeking training opportunities back home in OB-GYN, convinced me. He mentioned in passing that he had been accepted into a training program in Washington, D.C.

I immediately wrote to Dr. Moore, accepting his offer that would start in a couple of months. In the same letter, I asked if he could assist in getting Victoria a residency in pediatrics at the Boston Children's Hospital, part of the Harvard system and physically next to Brigham.

Dr. Moore's next letter arrived with news that Victoria had an appointment with the program director at the Children's Hospital a few days after our projected arrival. I liked the idea of going to Boston. Dr. Moore had mentioned the prospect of doing some research, which appealed to the inquisitive scientist in me. Did the letter seal our future in America?

31

PRIMARY FELLOWSHIP AGAIN

JUNE 1970

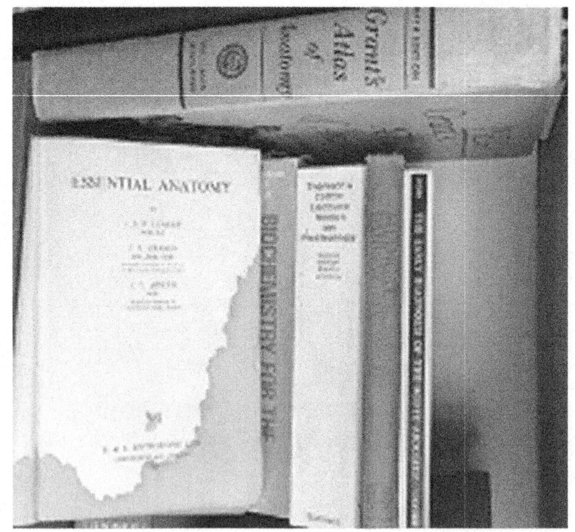

It's not about how bad you want it,
It's about how hard you are willing to work for it.
—Anonymous

It was now mid-April. The daffodils and crocuses peeked through the warming soil in Regent's Park, presaging spring—a new life, a new beginning. Our booking on the QE2 across the Atlantic to New York heralded a new start for me but particularly gave me another chance to become fully absorbed and engaged with the woman I had married. And Cunard's brochures showed passengers lounging on the deck sunning themselves. We would depart for Boston at the end of June 1970.

I had to pass the primary fellowship in surgery to redeem myself as a human being, free myself from self-loathing, and enhance my status across the pond. Having failed in my first attempt and accumulating some financial reserves working for ESSO, I signed up at the Royal College of Surgeons in Lincoln's Inn Fields to attend the several-week preparatory courses. I was embarking on a study marathon with potentially gratifying rewards: a surgical career, reaffirming my love for Victoria and rewarding us with a leisurely romantic holiday cruise—truthfully, the prospect of starting life over in Boston and the end of life with the temptations of Hanna.

The lectures were scheduled three times a week in the late afternoon. They covered anatomy, physiology and some pathology to a greater depth than we had studied in medical school, with an emphasis on practical knowledge and its application to patients. In anatomy—the structure related to function—lectures were given by the sage R. J. Last, Professor of Applied Anatomy. This elderly anatomist would gently walk on the stage, pick up some chalk, and draw a horizontal line on the blackboard. "What is this?"

The thirty-six students who sat riveted on the lecture benches yelled out various answers. He'd smile and say, "It's the base of the maxillary sinus," pointing to his face.

We immediately knew the topic he was teaching: the

anatomy of the head and neck. Proceeding from there, he'd draw additional lines and gradually, over the two hours, he'd build up, layer after layer, a three-dimensional view of the head with muscles, nerves and glands, continuing with the deep muscles of the neck including the salivary and lymph glands, all the while challenging his audience in a way that became a two-way conversation—funny, engaging, yet serious.

In another lecture covering sphincters, his question was simple. "What muscles do you use when pulling a rope?" The students shouted out several answers. He smiled, "The most important are the laryngeal muscles in your throat and your anal muscles; otherwise, you'd dump in your pants." We cheered. We got the point. We learned the lesson. How could one forget the information he elegantly imparted and so cleverly taught?

In contrast, the tall, portly, sagacious D. Slome, Professor of Applied Physiology, would strut onto the stage and enthusiastically engage us, teaching the basic concepts of physiology, embryology and the biochemical processes that applied to organs such as the liver. When it came to the diaphragm, he reminded us that during fetal development, it descended from the developing back muscles, and to emphasize the point, he dropped his spread handkerchief like a parachute. His lectures were permeated with such wisdom and witticisms that the audience became thoroughly engaged in his teachings and the material was enjoyable to learn.

Both professors were charming elderly showmen, skillful communicators and orators, stimulating their students. Neither one used slides or other visual aids. The two-hour lectures were a delight to attend. Not only did I learn the subjects effortlessly, but they became integrated into my surgical being.

Toward the end of the course, a young pathologist covered the most common diseases a surgeon was likely to encounter and the scientific basis for their treatment. The presentations were dry, earning the title "the science of suffering," where the students joked that we were the sufferers.

I knew that I was among the fortunate and privileged few who had insiders teaching and instructing us and was grateful that I could afford them. They gave me the direction and drive that encouraged me to maintain the discipline of study. After each lecture, I'd walk home singing and in good spirits, my head abuzz with surgically related matters. Perhaps, this time I might be among the lucky twenty percent to earn a passing grade.

Victoria was approaching the end of her second internship and was seldom at home. Gradually, I took over the flat, which began to resemble the cluttered rooms of my pre-A-level exam in Manchester and my tomb in Commonwealth Hall in the weeks before the second MB—notes and lists stuck on the mantel, pinned to the curtains and the bathroom mirror—lists in need of memorization and topics essential to study. Victoria was tolerant of the flat's transformation in the hope of my likely success.

During the last week, the material covered some exam subjects we might encounter, giving me a peek through a partially open door. Our lecturers had probably figured this out from the list of invited examiners and their known interests. Although I took note of these pointers, I was not a betting man and diligently learned everything, instilling a new confidence within me. I left the course with a feeling of optimism and excitement.

I felt thoroughly prepared and confident, yet the fear of failure lingered—my father's branding mark and my earlier sabotage of my own success. Early in June, wearing a dark gray suit bought from Moss Brothers using my ash cash, I walked briskly from Albany Street to the narrow back street basement entrance of Examination Hall. I noted that the location of the ventilation vent—where ten men had previously left their mark of anger and disappointment—was shielded.

Mr. Arthur Palmer once more directed me to a murmur-filled hall with examination desks. I took a seat among my fellow candidates. Face down in front of me lay an anatomy question sheet with a blank examination booklet for my answers. At 10 a.m., we were instructed to turn over the white sheet. The first question made me smile: "Describe the anatomy, relations, and blood supply of the left ureter." What a great question. This was the structure I had drawn on Victoria's abdomen some years ago. Was this a propitious omen? Several other questions followed, which I answered, finishing in time. After the lunch break, I faced the second written examination on applied physiology. Tired yet relaxed, I walked home in the late afternoon. I felt I had done well.

Victoria, who had completed her internship, took the last two weeks of June off as holiday. She was home and met me with a cup of tea. To remain in the present and to not disturb my equilibrium, I had asked her to keep our surroundings unchanged until I had the results. She had not attempted to gather up the books, my papers, or tidy up the notes that draped our breakfast table. Instead, she was busy packing two huge trunks in preparation for our sea voyage to New York.

"How was it?" she asked hesitantly.

"Interestingly, not as traumatic as the first time. I was able to answer all the questions thanks to the surgical courses," I replied. "But the tough exam, the *viva voce*, is the next hurdle."

"You'll do all right, I'm sure."

Exhausted, I fell into a deep sleep, snuggling with my wife in our cozy double bed.

Two days later, I entered the back of Examination Hall by the basement door once more, where I was met by Mr. Palmer asking for my candidate number.

"Twenty-four."

At my last try, Mr. Palmer seemed a man to be feared; now, he seemed quite amiable. He was small and well dressed, with keen insight into the stressed candidates and self-important judges, who were the examining surgeons. His skill of organizing the candidates for the orals was renowned. He gathered us into groups of twelve and reviewed the procedures. "When your number is called, go to your assigned cubicle. Each of the two examiners will question you for fifteen minutes. I will ring a bell, and you will move to the next cubicle. Should you perchance know the professor, excuse yourself and come see me. You will see another two groups in the afternoon." To reassure the candidates, he explained that the oral examiners were not those who had read our written answers and had no clue how well we had done.

At 10 a.m., the bell rang, and the first twelve candidates were directed by Mr. Palmer into their cubicles. A calm thirty minutes later, our group filed toward the front of the firing line. Sitting down, I was asked my number, and after a polite greeting, I faced my first question.

"What is a sphincter?"

"It's an area of high pressure surrounding a cylindrical structure such as the orbicularis oris, the larynges, the esophagus and the anal sphincter, controlled by slings of muscles."

"Would you consider the pylorus in the duodenum a sphincter?" he retorted.

"Indeed."

"And how would you describe its function?"

I was fully in the present and totally engaged by this question and the numerous others that followed. His partner took over and fired his questions at me. My responses were cogent and in depth. Unaware of the passing of time, when the bell rang, I was reluctant to leave; I was enjoying facing the challenges thrown at me and sharing the information I had acquired. I moved to the next cubicle, feeling in high spirits, like a boxer eager to step into another ring. The whole process was repeated when I faced a new pair of professors and a new set of anatomy questions.

By late morning, I faced the physiology *viva voce*. Once more, I felt confident and answered convincingly. The questions given to me ranged from cardiac output to the amount of bile the liver produces after receiving one unit of whole blood. I knew the answers.

Generally, when a candidate had done well or was borderline and there were a few minutes left in the interrogation, the professors might challenge him—either to determine the limits of the candidate's knowledge or perhaps to throw a lifebuoy question. So, I was caught off guard when I was next asked, "What do you think causes birth defects in infants born with shortened limbs?"

I interpreted the question to mean that I must be a borderline candidate, and I wanted to yell, "No, no, please ask me a surgically relevant one; give me another chance, I have a few minutes left." Panic welled up from deep within me. Sensing my hesitation and perhaps my alarm, he suggested several probabilities to which I answered monosyllabically. The bell rang. With that I left, now uncertain of my performance.

Per Mr. Palmer's instructions, at around 4 p.m. we crowded into a stuffy, windowless room and sat in various states of anxiety, pondering our fate. Had I just wasted six months of study, or had I made the grade? Fifteen minutes later, Mr. Palmer appeared at the door, list in hand. Silence fell upon the wretched crowd.

In a deep baritone voice, he declared, "I will read out the number of only successful candidates. Please step forward. I will ask you if you are 'Dr. So-and-So,' and when you acknowledge your name, I will tell you, 'Congratulations Mr. So-and-So,' indicating, as you step through the door, that you are on your way to becoming a surgeon."

Raising his paper, he read the first number, "Candidate number three." There were moans and a yelp of joy as the successful doctor rose and approached Mr. Palmer. And so it went down the line, the announced numbers approaching closer and closer to the twenties. My heart started to race and my gray suit became a tightly fitting sweat suit. My body perspired profusely.

I could hardly breath as Mr. Palmer voiced ". . . numbers nineteen, twenty, twenty-one." The run of successful candidates preceding my number surely meant that the next few numbers were those of failed candidates, to obey the law of averages. Mr. Palmer shuffled his papers and continued, "Number twenty-four, twenty-five . . ." The immense relief I felt hearing that I had passed nearly led to a meltdown. I rose on wobbly legs, gathered myself together, and numbly strode to the front door.

"Dr. Meguid?"

"Yes."

"Congratulations, Mr. Meguid." And with a wave of his hand, he ushered me out into the cool day—now a man reborn.

I started to run down the street through the light rain when a taxi appeared in the middle of the one-way road. I hailed it, aware that another man on the opposite pavement had hailed it, too. The taxi stopped in the middle of the street. I ran for it and opened the door at the same time as the other man. I got in first, so technically, it was mine. As I looked across the cab, I recognized one of my examiners. I graciously relented and exited. The taxi took off, leaving me standing in the rain.

Resuming my trot toward Albany Street, I realized the drops running down my face were a mixture of heaven's rain and my tears of joy, for I had achieved my first goal to become a surgeon. But they were also the shedding of tears of self-pity and anger at the persistent shadow of my dead father—the man who was never satisfied by what I had achieved as a child and who had been perpetually disappointed in me during the few years we had together. They were tears of contrition for my selfish behavior, for the pain I had inflicted on Hanna, tears for the pain I would have caused Victoria and tears for the relief of overcoming my pain of abandonment and tears of joy for finally having passed.

Continuing my dash home to Victoria, and in a hoarse voice, I yelled out repeatedly, "I did it. I PASSED. I PASSED." Passersby in Gower and Euston Streets must have thought I was an escaped mental case. And, in a way, I was.

I had done it. Despite my parents or maybe because of them, I was standing on the initial rung of the ladder to mastering the scalpel in earnest and becoming a surgeon. Nothing would stop me now.

And in the doorway stood Victoria. "Did you fail?"

"Passed," I said hugging her. "One of only twenty percent."

"Then why are you crying?"

I did not answer. I had many reasons to weep.

32

ADIEU BUT NOT GOODBYE

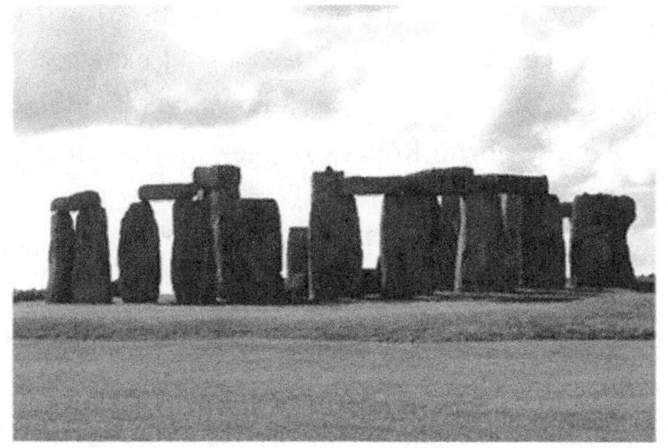

Love is the only thing you get more of by giving it away.
—Tom Wilson

We had two weeks to pack up, do our rounds of family farewells, and return the flat key to our landlord before we boarded Cunard's pride, the QE2. On Tuesday June 30, we would set sail from Southampton to New York. We didn't have a crystal-clear idea as to how long we'd be in Boston, but expected to be there between one and three years.

Victoria had started to pack our things into one of the aluminum sea trunks. I collected my medical books, folders of notes, and my precious Royal College lecture summaries and placed them into the second chest. She stood beside me as I kneeled arranging the weighty material like a big puzzle at the bottom of the steamer trunk.

"Do you still need these? They are quite heavy and you've passed the exam," Victoria said.

She was right, to a point. I checked myself. Surely, I could chuck them out. I had integrated the material into my surgical being. Yet, I felt as dependent on the information as a patient who hangs on their physician's every word.

"Yes, I want them. It's too soon for me to throw them out." They were my comfort notes—my Plan B. I expected to return to London to sit for my final fellowship examination and become a Fellow of the Royal College—the esteemed surgical qualification and key to our future.

"That was just a thought," she said. "I'm not taking my books with me."

"You're smarter than me. Once I've got my final fellowship, then perhaps I'll chuck them—you know how I feel about discarding papers, any papers. Anyway, I may need the notes to brush up before the next exam."

Our implied conversation was based on my assumption that we would return to London. We'd settle down, I pursuing my career at a teaching hospital such as University College and she her pediatrics, until we planned to have offspring. I removed the endless to-do lists tacked onto the curtains, the memory lists taped to the mantelpiece and bathroom mirror, that had converted our small flat into a paper jungle. After sorting them out, these too were placed in what was now designated as my trunk.

The activities moved along at varying speeds, depending on fatigue and mood. Certainly, Victoria was less tired than I was for she had completed her house jobs by early June at a time I was making my run for a slide into the surgical world.

We were both buoyant at completing an important stage of life and starting out on a new phase. I looked forward to our life in Boston, learning innovative operations, and being with Victoria, but most of all to get away from the person I had become—thoughts of the past year as I stared out of the window. I knew it was the pain of my deception and double life, my fear of loneliness, that invoked a physical flashback to the helpless four-year-old boy abandoned in Germany.

"Are you alright?"

"Yes, yes," I said forcefully, and then as an afterthought, "Just apprehensive of the uncertainty that lies ahead of us."

"Scary. But we'll be all right."

"We'll be together," I added.

I rose from my kneeling and we embraced. "We'll be together," I whispered again.

Together was the "now" word. I was with Victoria all the time.

We planned together.

Packed together.

Dined at the Agra together.

Said our goodbyes to Mr. Subhan Sultan together.

Rested together.

And made love, together.

Gradually, like a growing plant, our new tender twigs intertwined as I bent toward Victoria's light, and I saw again the woman I first fell in love with.

As the flat took on an air of normalcy, certain pieces of furniture, items we had borrowed from Shirley and Victoria's grandmother, Dagmar, had to be returned. Several boxes of our stuff needed storage with family and friends until our return.

We packed a rented van, and drove south of London in glorious sunshine, swathed in the mood of victorious conquerors through Surry to Haslemere arriving in time for lunch. Dagmar, who was quite elderly, lived in two old shepherds' cottages renovated into one, which retained low doorways and ceilings, small windows, large fireplaces at each end of the dim living room and squeaking wooden floors in the upstairs bedrooms. Victoria smiled a wicked smile as she whispered that Dagmar had the squeaky boards put in so she could tell which guest was slipping from one bedroom to another. And with that she winked at me.

Sitting outside, we ate slowly, having no self-imposed deadlines, basking in the early summer sunlight and surrounded by Dagmar's exquisite English garden. Lunch was tasty and as meager as her £5 marriage gift. We dropped off a table and said our farewells. Both Victoria and I, as well as Dagmar, sensed the hint that this goodbye might well be the last one.

We resumed our drive south, heading to college friends near Lymington where we were expected for tea. The mood in the van had changed. "That was very nice," I said. "I do hope we will see her again on our return," wondering if Victoria shared my sentiments.

"Well, she's quite old. When I used to stay with her, we shared a bedroom and I'd listen to her breathing at night, fearful it might stop."

"I know what you mean. It's frightening. I too was very fretful when Oma broke her hip and I wasn't allowed to see her. Later, I often dreamt she had died." She gazed at me as I added, "Of course it was my Dad who went and did that."

"You believe that?"

"What?" I said as I maneuvered the narrow road with its increased afternoon traffic.

"That he willed to die?"

"I thought so. For a long time, I believed that he only died to punish me."

"Really?"

"Well, probably not really," I admitted.

The van was several pounds lighter after we dropped boxes of books and other nonessentials with our friends for storage. This time we said "adieu," for our friends were working for companies that had connections overseas and it would only be a matter of time before they'd be our guests on the other side of the pond.

Fortified by a sumptuous tea, I drove as Victoria navigated our way to the Lymington car ferry. I relished her company, her closeness, the air she exuded. "It's been a hard day's night, and I've been working like a dog," I sang, and not knowing the rest of the lyrics I continued to chant "dara ra, dara da, daram dum." She joined in. "When I get home to you, I'll find the things that you do," and we sang in chorus as I squeezed her thigh, "Will make me feel all right."

We felt very special. We both were registered physicians in England—real doctors. Furthermore, I now stood on the first rung of becoming a surgeon, a person who is given the trust to pick up a knife and cut into a fellow human with the intent of healing them. I felt the silent pride, even the quiet hubris, that Mr. Kingdom, Desmond and Mr. Maingot projected with a degree of confidence. This was contentment after the stormy period when I felt disconnected from reality, life and Victoria.

The car ferry cut through the Solent, heading east away from the low setting sun as we headed to Cowes, where we disembarked. We arrived in Seaview in the last of the day's waning light. Shirley was delighted to see us. Her mood was on the upside, cheerful to see her daughter and glad for the return of her armchair. A home cooked dinner was ready.

"Must you go already darling?" Shirley said, almost pleading after we'd spent three days with her. "Can't you stay a few more days? You're going to go all the way to Boston and I won't see you in forever so long."

"It's only for a couple of years, Mummy. I'm sure we will come and visit. Or you'll be our guest in Boston," Victoria reassured. "In the few days we have left we'd like to take your car for a day and do some sightseeing. Visit Stonehenge and Salisbury Cathedral and be alone together. And we still have more to pack, there are so many things to still do."

"Darling, you know how down I get when you leave."

I thought of how Sheik Amin wept when I left his company, tears that had at first mystified me, but with progressing age I began to understand their meaning. His tears and his repeated imploring for me to stay longer when I announced that I had to leave took the "well" out of my farewell.

"You have your friends at the Yacht Club. We'll only be a couple of days then I'll be back to go with you to your GP before we leave," Victoria said encouragingly.

Packing a hamper into the car, we crossed the Solent once more on another joyous blue-sky day. An aura of love and hope pervaded Shirley's comfortable car. We leisurely meandered north and soon reached the New Forest—the largest remaining tracts of heathland and forest in southern England. Rolling down the windows, we inhaled and relished the rich scents of nature emitted by the damp earth, the fresh scent of heather, and the sweet and woody smell of the ferns that carpeted the landscape. Rays of sunlight peeking through the canopy of oaks, elm and sweet chestnut played patterns in the dim undergrowth. From time to time, we saw deer and donkeys. The utter peace was occasionally pierced by a woodlark. The forest reminded me of the more pleasant times during my preteenage youth in Germany—the spring mushroom hunts with

Oma and the summer swims *au naturel* in the large fish pond of Rissen where a gang of boys had cycled and dared each other to strip.

Neither the stolen kiss nor my caressing the nape of Victoria's neck sufficed in toning down our ardor. I turned into a gravel track and found a secluded spot far from the road where we rolled out a blanket and lay silently on our backs gazing into the void above us listening to the call of a forest warbler.

We rested. We rested in silence. It was the first time in a long time . . . perhaps in years . . . so long that I couldn't remember that we were truly alone. Alone, by ourselves to connect to our inner selves, to our inner deep self, independent of thought and action or even the presence or influence of the other. The silence of nature sounded Elysian, like the silent sound I experienced in the pinnacle of meditation when gliding, rowing and focused on surgery. The engrossed inner solitude that spins out the center into pin point peripheral. In this silent, dark world, my misdeed was obvious—I had hurt and betrayed my wife.

Resting my cheek on her bared soft abdomen and embracing it—the anatomy I worshipped, I heard Victoria's muffled voice. "What are you doing? We're in public." She adjusted the blanket to cover my head, uneasy what this was leading to. I hugged her belly. In mute communion with her tummy, silently tears rolled down my cheeks and onto the midriff, pooling in the well of her belly button and gently running down its sides. The weeping of regret was more open —less controlled.

I whispered, "I'm so sorry. I wasn't trying to hurt you."

After a silence, I raised my head and blew my nose. We looked at each other, both propped up on our elbows. "Don't let it happen again. Betrayal hurts. I hope this is the end between you and Magdalena."

Victoria's eyes were soft. Leaning over, I touched her face, her hair, and tasted her lips. Dare I let my hands stray. She shivered. I felt her heartbeat and while the tree canopy parted, we savored ecstasy. Lying beside her. gazing at the treetops, and the occasional rays of direct sunlight, I couldn't understand what had made me stray.

Turning to me, Victoria asked in a quiet voice, "What are you thinking about?"

"Oh. A Sanskrit poem I once learned. It's on the essence of love that gives meaning to us, to our relationship, to you my dearest wife."

"Tell me. Can you recite it for me?"

"I'll try. *Panting and pale from Love, Then from your cheeks my love, Scent of sweat, I love, And when our bodies love, Now to relax in love, After the stress of love, Ever still more I love, Our mingled breath of love.*"

"Oh, that was so nice. When did you learn that?"

"In Manchester, after I failed the lower sixth and I had to repeat it but this time with an emphasis in biology and general knowledge. I had a friend. David was his name. We became close . . . almost like brotherly love."

"Do you still know him?"

"Sort of. He went to Liverpool Medical School and then we lost touch. He was a sensitive, gentle type. He loved music and poetry. He'd come over to visit in secret."

"In secret? Why? What do you mean? What are you telling me?" her face frowned.

"No, it's not what you think," I said, taking her hand and explaining that he was raised in a strict Jewish home and sort of rebelled. "He'd spend a few hours with me and we would play LPs of Johnny Mathis. Anyway, he had a poetry book that he lent to me. That's where I first read the poem."

Victoria relaxed once more. "Was he nice?"

"Yes. I loved him like a brother."

"Where is he now? Can we meet him?"

"I think in Israel. But if he is in New York, then we'll likely meet him."

"Hungry?"

We rose.

As we traveled the A303 north Stonehenge rose impressively out of Salisbury Plain. Hand in hand we ambled up the grassy incline toward the thirteen-foot-tall prehistoric monument. We marveled at the concentric ring of massive stones. I touched the rough stone almost as awestruck as I had been when first climbing the great pyramid of Cheops. We sat on the grass and Victoria read from the tour guide. "Carbon dating of skeleton remains found in several hundred burial mounds surrounding this iconic structure suggest it was built during the Stone age. The original purpose of Stonehenge is unclear. Some have speculated that it was a temple made for the worship of ancient earth deities, while some describe it as a burial site." The description that made more sense to me was that it was an astrological observatory to allow study of the sun and moon because the stones line up with the summer and winter solstice, similar to the ancient Egyptian temple of Abu Simbel.

The view of nearby Salisbury Cathedral from afar was majestic. Victoria knew of John Constable's paintings and insisted we first meander to the meadow to glimpse it from there. We sat in silence on our blanket and ate our sandwiches, absorbing the peace of the pastoral landscape before enjoying the grandeur of the Gothic spire.

With barely a week left, we departed the Isle of Serenity and returned to London to find our elderly landlord sorry to see that we would be leaving.

"Now that you are both doctors would you be interested in acquiring the entire terrace house?"

"How much?"

"I'd like to get £6,000."

£6,000 for a house in Regent's Park, almost in Central London? My first thought was that we didn't have such funds and I wondered if Shirley would have helped. We'd have an ideal home.

The die was cast. Boston was our next destination. I was glad we were leaving London behind us.

33

ATLANTIC BREEZE

A journey of one thousand miles begins with one step.
—Lao Tzu

The QE2 was a classic beauty, the majestic, elegantly designed flagship of the Cunard Line, built with speed and luxury in mind, in contrast to the sturdy Esperia that had taken me from Egypt. Unlike the Italian ship, where the barriers between the class grades were ambiguous, in the QE2 they were distinct. We paid £600 for the five-day transatlantic cruise to New York in a third-class cabin, funds we drew from Mr. Winterberry's reserve, my first surgical patient, who had turned my £5 weekly food allowance into a small fortune only six years ago—a gamble I never regretted.

We departed England with our two sea trunks in late June on a perfectly beautiful summer's day. Contrary to Shirley's dark prediction, she was upbeat, cheerful, and exuberant when we met her with Mother and Auntie Jo on the docks at Southampton. A band played beside the ship, adding a festive mood even before we boarded. We were greeted by the social director on embarking. Victoria stayed on deck with our guests sipping free champagne.

Seeking our tourist-class cabin, a steward led me to a set of spiraling steps that descended, to my dismay, to a lower and lower and lower deck where the ship's engine vibrations became progressively louder. Finally, on Deck 1, he opened the door on a small, dim, and windowless interior cabin.

"Surely this is a mistake," I said indignantly. "We are two doctors going on our honeymoon. I really need a window. Can't you do better?"

The old Egyptian tradition of baksheesh came in handy. The steward checked his clipboard, swiveled in the narrow passageway, and flung open a door on the opposite side. The cabin was large and roomy, had two portholes, two single beds pushed together, and a walk-in shower.

"Fantastic."

Our guests departed in the late afternoon in a cascade of streamers and confetti. At the rail, with the sun sinking behind England, a cool breeze rose to chill us. I put my arm about Victoria's waist and drew her close. Together, Victoria and I had each completed six years of extraordinary stress and almost continuous study—most of it as two individuals. It transformed us from high school pupils to young doctors—in my case, a surgeon. At the rail we were one, comforting each other at the rupture of the ties in our lives.

We waved goodbye as tugboats slowly pulled the QE2 into the Thames. The deep resonant farewell horn mixed with the strains of "Auld Lang Syne," which wafted in the cool evening breeze. The graying figures continued to wave endless goodbyes while they became smaller and smaller in the shadow of the afternoon sun.

We persisted waving too, for we didn't want our bonds with England to weaken. The ship steamed into the English Channel toward France on its way to America.

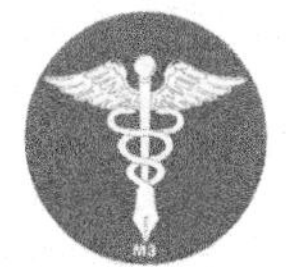

ACKNOWLEDGMENTS

Writing is a lonely task but a book requires the help of others. Loving thanks to the family and friends who have generously provided assistance, editing and encouragement in completing this book including Ellen Lesser, Lori Handelman, Jennifer Brice, Joan Gerberding, Martin Gillieson, Rory McCloy, and Jo-Ann Sanborn. As always, my gratitude to Carolyn Ring who once again took a manuscript and made it into a book. Lucy, my faithful Chihuahua sat by my side throughout the years of writing A *Surgeon's Tale.*

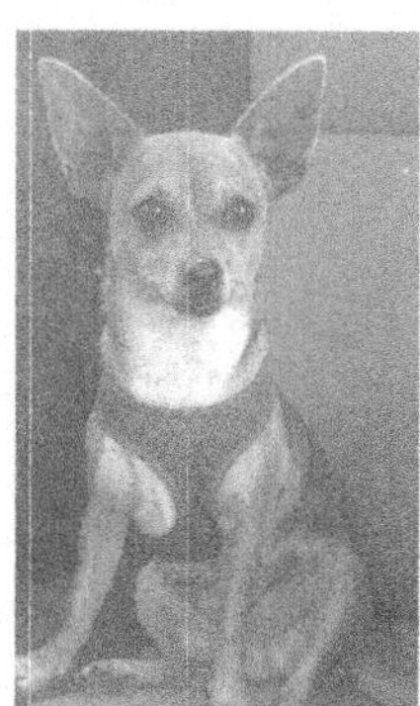

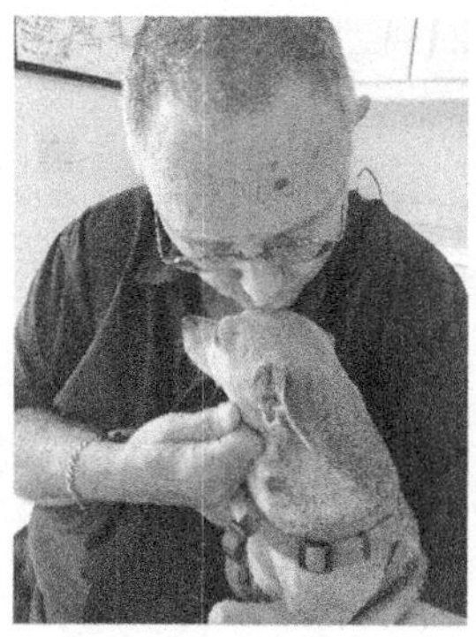

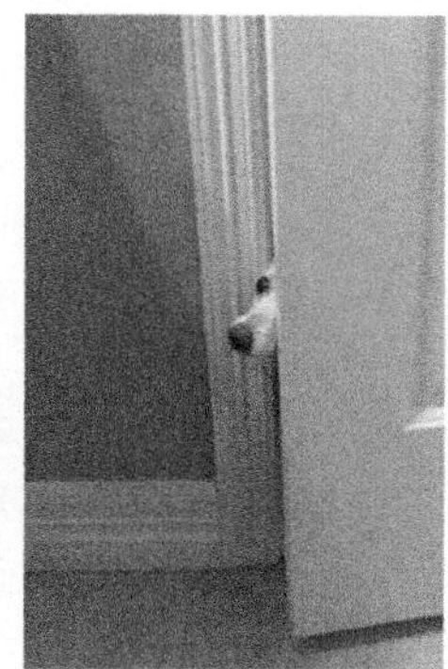

Please visit my website for more information including trailers and videos about the previous books in this series. Lucy and I would love to hear from you. Sign the pop-up if you'd like to hear from me regularly.

www.michaelmeguid.com

ABOUT THE AUTHOR

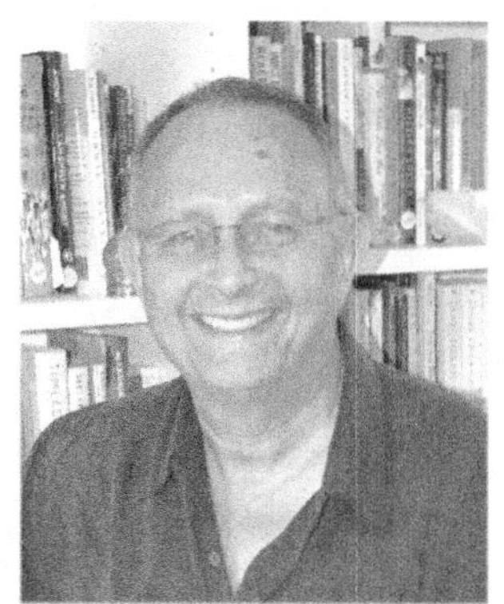

Michael M. Meguid is a creative nonfiction writer, surgeon and researcher who blends his learnings from each walk of life into a series called *A Surgeon's Tale*, a historical biography that reaches beyond the merely personal to convey something of the cultures, people, politics and places that touch the inscrutable heart of human nature.

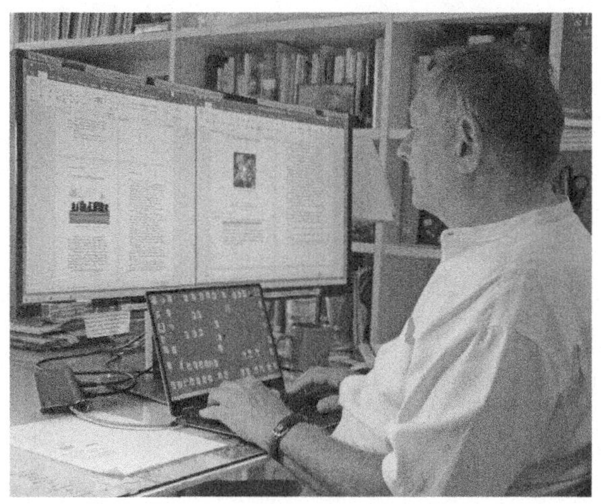

GREAT JOY, GREAT SORROW

Please enjoy an excerpt from Michael M. Meguid's fourth biographical novel, *Great Joy, Great Sorrow*, which will be released in early 2022.

LEROY THE INVISIBLE

I caught up with my residents as they hurriedly pushed the gurney with a combative young man into the OR. All they had told me over the phone, shortly after 4 a.m., was that an eighteen-year-old man had slipped off a third-floor window ledge while trying to break into an apartment some thirty minutes earlier. He was now in profound shock, running a low blood pressure from a presumed life-threatening internal hemorrhage. They'd meet me in the OR. Within minutes, I was speeding down the Mass Pike to Boston City Hospital, fueled by an adrenaline rush.

As with all such blunt abdominal cases where major internal bleeding is suspected, few invasive or radiological tests had been done. The one quick, on-the-spot test my residents did in the ER—the semi-quantitative newsprint test—was positive. In this test, a needle attached to IV tubing and 500ml of saline is stuck into the lower abdominal midline. The entire volume is rapidly run into the abdominal cavity, and then the bag is lowered so that the saline siphons back into the plastic bag. If the return-fluid is sufficiently turbid with blood so that newsprint cannot be read through it, research shows that the results highly correlate with bleeding from a major internal organ such as the liver. The key is to get the patient to the OR as quickly as possible, open up the abdomen, and take care of the injury to stop the hemorrhage before the patient bleeds to death.

LeRoy lay naked on the gurney, and I saw with envy that he had a fine ebony physique; in contrast, my body showed the signs of physical neglect. He was very muscular, with a thick neck from lifting weights, and well-developed shoulders and arms. He had the classic six-pack abdomen. He had obviously spent much time body building. I wished I had such a body; instead, I'd spent my time building my mind. Several large-bore IVs had been stuck into his arms and were wide open, as fluids poured into his veins trying to keep pace with his bleeding, supporting his low blood pressure. The Foley catheter in his bladder drained cloudy yellow urine, suggestive of blood, and maybe an injury to his kidneys. His youthful body shimmered in the OR light. His belly was distended.

He was inadequately sedated, thrashing and restless, fighting his endotracheal tube which was providing 100% oxygen to his lungs. He tugged at his restrained arms. Our eyes met—a wild and frightened stare. Reading his mind, I too wondered if he'd make it. Abruptly, his head and arms slumped as the anesthetist gave him a slug of a sedative. As we cautiously moved him onto the OR table, I saw that he had a grossly disfigured, twisted left thigh bone from a fractured femur. He was bleeding into his thigh, which was tense and double its usual size, shining with a bluish hue from accumulated blood.

Without scrubbing, I gowned and gloved. The circulating nurse poured a bottle of antiseptic Betadine over his abdomen, which ran down the sides of his belly and dripped onto the floor. She secured the "seat belt" over his good right leg and cradled his fractured leg in pillows. The orthopedic resident was on his way to see the fracture and the hastily obtained ER X-ray of his twisted leg, while the anesthetist was fretting about his continued low blood pressure, egging me on and calling out for more units of blood. Together with my resident, we rapidly draped his torso, the wet Betadine soaking through the water-proof drapes and the front of my gown, into my underpants stinging my balls, and dripping into my shoes. We worked feverishly against time.

Shortly before 5 a.m., I hesitated for a very brief moment, scalpel in hand, reluctant to place a scar through his beautiful abdominal wall. Then I made a single, swift, full thickness midline incision through his hairless skin—one bold slash with the knife into his abdominal cavity from xyphoid to pubis. Stem to stern, straight through his belly button.

I expected to find lots of free blood, a fractured liver or spleen, or ruptured vessels—usual injuries associated with a fall from a significant height. I found . . . nothing!

Nothing. There was no free blood in his abdomen, and his organs were all intact

LeRoy's shock was from the profuse bleeding into the muscles of his thigh, tracking up the retroperitoneal space at the back of his pelvis and up into his lower back, pushing the roots of his guts forward, where some blood seeped through from the back into the abdominal cavity. It was barely sufficient to have given a positive newsprint test. Could the intern in the ER have over-interpreted the degree of blood in the return?

The orthopedic attending and his entourage of residents and medical students trooped into the OR and questioned our findings. I could only shake my head. Suspecting that I was overlooking an injury, I systematically re-examined his entire abdomen: every single organ, his liver, spleen, stomach, pancreas, the small and large bowel, his major vessels, his kidneys and bladder, every organ between his diaphragm and his pelvic floor—at a more deliberate and measured pace, taking my time to be absolutely sure I was not overlooking a subtle injury.

Again, I found no internal injuries.

Without question, the source of his bleeding was the broken femoral shaft bone, a very vascular structure. The adrenaline rush drained out of me. Suddenly I felt deflated and tired. *But I was glad for LeRoy.* What had been a close call was over. He was now going to live. He was now going to make it. LeRoy was going to recover; he was going to go home. But at the same time, it was unfortunate that I had scarred his body with the standard trauma-type slash incision with the intention of saving his life.

After closing his belly, I scrubbed out and the orthopedic surgeon moved in to fix his fractured leg and stop the bleeding bone. Protocol dictated that LeRoy became their patient and he was transferred to the care of the orthopedic service as we bowed out.

By noon, LeRoy had been moved to the ICU, where he lay in the first bed by the door. During the next few weeks, I saw him at least twice a day as I passed him on my way through the ICU to see my patients during my early morning and late evening rounds.

One day, after thirty days, his bed was empty.

"Where is LeRoy?"

"Dead," was the reply.

LeRoy had died?

"Yes. This morning."

I was stunned. How could an eighteen-year-old physically fit human specimen just die from a broken leg? I went into the bowels of Boston City Hospital where medical records were kept and reviewed his hospital records. The records showed he had no signs of other injuries.

On admission, LeRoy had weighed 150 pounds. He lost

almost 34 pounds during his thirty-day hospital stay. Although the order was written for an oral diet, his records showed that he had eaten very little; no calorie counts had been noted to record whether he ate and how much he consumed. He had essentially been maintained on an intravenous drip of 5% glucose-saline. One liter provides fifty grams of glucose, or barely two teaspoons of sugar—the equivalent of 170 calories. He had received three liters a day, getting a total of approximately six teaspoons of sugar—510 calories, or about two candy bars a day for thirty days.

To survive his massive leg injury, the insult of the shock from the bleeding, plus the stress of two major operations, he would need at least 3000 calories per day. Not just as glucose, but also as protein, vitamins, trace elements and minerals to permit healing of his injured tissues. In the absence of intense nutritional support, his muscles broke down to provide his daily nutrient needs. When he ran out of his critical muscle mass, LeRoy died.

He died in a Harvard University hospital from malnutrition.

The date was August 1976.

To this day, I wonder whether his death certificate truly reflected the cause of death: hospital-related malnutrition! Four years earlier, the *Boston Globe* had run a headline: "Patients in a Harvard Hospital Become Malnourished." A young surgeon had conducted a study of the nutritional status of general surgical patients in a particular Harvard hospital and published a paper in the prestigious peer-reviewed *Journal of the American Medical Association*. It revealed that fifteen percent of surgical patients were already malnourished on admission. But worse, the frequency of malnutrition rose to sixty percent after fourteen days in the hospital. This increased the death rate three-fold.

The results hit the proud Boston surgical community like a bombshell, especially the great and powerful men of the

Harvard surgical world, the very men who were our surgical teachers, and mentors—the surgical power brokers of the time, whose disciples we were, and on whose coattails our careers were riding. They took great umbrage at the suggestion that under their impeccable surgical care, in these hallowed Harvard halls, the incidence of malnutrition increased. It implied gross neglect!

I was in the research lab at Harvard studying nutrition and metabolism when the proverbial shit hit the fan. The *Globe*'s story was the buzz throughout the hospital, the Harvard medical community, and all of Boston. I kept my head down as the ferocious fury raged about me, and veiled threats were heaped on this poor young surgeon. His academic career was stalled for decades, until those slighted ultimately passed on.

At the time of LeRoy's death, I felt a pang of guilt, because barely six weeks previously I'd started my first job. Not only was I LeRoy's surgeon, but on the basis of my limited experience in the research lab I was appointed Head of the Surgical Clinical Nutrition Team.

The team consisted of several persons with specialized skills. The dietitian was well-versed in recognizing and diagnosing specific nutritional problems as they related to the patient's disease or those induced by the stress of their therapy during their hospital stay. The nurse was familiar with the various intravenous catheters and nasogastric tubes, their placement and their daily care, for, if infected, these catheters could become a source of infection. Finally, the team had a pharmacist who was familiar with the sterile compounding of the various nutrients, vitamins, minerals and trace elements, and their compatibility.

In sum, these individuals reflected a highly skilled group of health care personnel who prevented and treated malnutrition. The problem with malnutrition was that its presence in addition to a disease increased hospital-related infection from fifteen to seventy percent. It also increased the death rate threefold. The traditional way was for a physician to consult me when recognizing his patient had a nutritional problem. However, since nutrition was not taught in medical schools or during residency, many physicians didn't recognize a nutrition-related problem. I realized this was a system failure. I had to institute a hospital-wide policy whereby patients at risk of nutritional problems would automatically be brought to the team's attention for treatment.

I could see that this would involve several delicate issues: turf, propriety of the doctor-patient relationship, relinquishing care on one aspect of care to an uninvited team, and maybe even slighting another surgeon by implication, because it acknowledged the failure to recognize "malnutrition." I sensed that if I was to institute such an early warning system, I'd have to recruit the help of a senior surgeon with authority and standing among the faculty, so that this would not be seen as "an upstart's scheme to drum up business." Despite my efforts during my time at Boston City Hospital, I was unable to institute policy whereby each patient was nutritionally assessed by the team on admission and if found at risk of malnutrition, the team would automatically and without a formal consult intervene upon the patient's behalf. It wasn't until a number of years later that Title 22 mandated such a practice.

Nutrition research at the time of LeRoy's death tended to focus on animal husbandry. Making chickens breasts larger and pigs and cattle grow faster seemed to be the priorities. There were two *human* nutrition departments, nationwide. One was at MIT across the Charles River, and the other was at UCLA across the country. Having a young family and having to earn my living as an operating surgeon, my choice was easy.

My inquiries to MIT in August 1978 led to an invitation for an interview with the department head, on a Saturday night, his place: his end-of-summer departmental party. The gist of our conversation—under a clear, starry canopy, poolside, with lit candles floating on the pool and soft music in the background—was that MIT's Department of Nutrition and Food Science needed a physician to supervise ongoing human nutrition studies in healthy MIT students. Was I interested? If so, I could then also attend classes to meet the nutrition "course requirements."

I agreed.

What a deal! I was going to get the knowledge that I needed to bolster my title-ordained authority, and that I wanted to better treat my patients, just by keeping a periodic eye on young, healthy kids. It was a piece of cake. Somehow, I had missed the significance of the code words "course requirements."

It rang no alarm bells, and held no masochistic connotations of graduate courses, lectures, term papers, deadlines, or exams, until a few days later when the MIT admissions officer frantically called me to come promptly and complete a set of forms, because the winter term was about to start.

So, at the age of thirty-five, after four years of college, five years of medical school, and seven years of surgical training, I sat once more with twenty-two-year-old super-smart kids in a classroom. I was draped over my desk, going to classes in the morning at MIT, doing my elective operations in the afternoon at Boston City Hospital, and often operating at night on emergencies. At such times I felt bedraggled and sleep-deprived. Did I really want to do this? I felt like a misfit as various teachers droned on and on and on about nutrition. My pager, akin to a live grenade, was dangling from my belt threatening to go off at any moment. I hoped and prayed that it wouldn't, so I could remain as inconspicuous as possible.

Thus, I lived the double life of an authoritative surgeon on one side of the Charles and a humble, exhausted and insecure graduate student on the other bank. During three challenging years I completed the graduate courses and attained the knowledge of human nutrition that would become complementary to my surgery. Now I could treat my cancer patients while providing them with intensive nutritional support and prevent them from becoming malnourished.

For oft, while on my couch I lie,
In vacant or in pensive mood,
LeRoy flashes on my inward eye,
I see his face, again.
Our eyes meet once more.
They are soft and forgiving.

And as his image fades, I whisper, as if to a sleeping child, "My blessings and gratitude to LeRoy for having helped so many other patients."

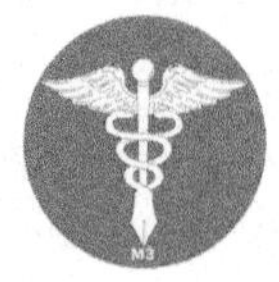

Made in United States
North Haven, CT
01 October 2022